T0321037

Computational
Blood Cell Mechanics

Chapman & Hall/CRC Mathematical and Computational Biology

About the Series

This series aims to capture new developments and summarise what is known over the entire spectrum of mathematical and computational biology and medicine. It seeks to encourage the integration of mathematical, statistical, and computational methods into biology by publishing a broad range of textbooks, reference works, and handbooks. The titles included in the series are meant to appeal to students, researchers, and professionals in the mathematical, statistical, and computational sciences and fundamental biology and bioengineering, as well as interdisciplinary researchers involved in the field. The inclusion of concrete examples and applications and programming techniques and examples is highly encouraged.

Series Editors

Xihong Lin
Mona Singh
N. F. Britton
Anna Tramontano
Maria Victoria Schneider
Nicola Mulder

Chromatin: Structure, Dynamics, Regulation
Ralf Blossey

Mathematical Models of Plant-Herbivore Interactions
Zhilan Feng, Donald DeAngelis

Computational Exome and Genome Analysis
Peter N. Robinson, Rosario Michael Piro, Marten Jager

Gene Expression Studies Using Affymetrix Microarrays
Hinrich Gohlmann, Willem Talloen

Big Data in Omics and Imaging
Association Analysis
Momiao Xiong

Introduction to Proteins
Structure, Function, and Motion, Second Edition
Amit Kessel, Nir Ben-Tal

Big Data in Omics and Imaging
Integrated Analysis and Causal Inference
Momiao Xiong

Computational Blood Cell Mechanics
Road Towards Models and Biomedical Applications
Ivan Cimrák, Iveta Jančigová

For more information about this series please visit: https://www.crcpress.com/ Chapman--HallCRC-Mathematical-and-Computational-Biology/book-series/ CHMTHCOMBIO

Computational
Blood Cell Mechanics
Road Towards Models and
Biomedical Applications

Ivan Cimrák

Iveta Jančigová

Department of Software Technologies

Faculty of Management Science and Informatics

University of Žilina

Slovakia

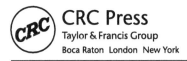

CRC Press

Taylor & Francis Group

Boca Raton London New York

CRC Press is an imprint of the
Taylor & Francis Group, an **informa** business

A CHAPMAN & HALL BOOK

CRC Press
Taylor & Francis Group
6000 Broken Sound Parkway NW, Suite 300
Boca Raton, FL 33487-2742

© 2019 by Taylor & Francis Group, LLC
CRC Press is an imprint of Taylor & Francis Group, an Informa business

No claim to original U.S. Government works

Printed on acid-free paper
Version Date: 20180813

International Standard Book Number-13: 978-1-138-50608-4 (Hardback)

Library of Congress Cataloging-in-Publication Data

Names: Cimrak, Ivan, author. | Jancigova, Iveta, author.
Title: Computational blood cell mechanics : road towards models and
biomedical applications / Ivan Cimrak, Iveta Jancigova.
Description: Boca Raton, Fla. : CRC Press, 2018.
Identifiers: LCCN 2018024673| ISBN 9781138506084 (hardback : alk. paper) |
ISBN 9781315146775 (ebook)
Subjects: LCSH: Blood cells. | Blood--Research. | Computational biology.
Classification: LCC QP94 .C56 2018 | DDC 612.1/1--dc23
LC record available at https://lccn.loc.gov/2018024673

Visit the Taylor & Francis Web site at
http://www.taylorandfrancis.com

and the CRC Press Web site at
http://www.crcpress.com

*To you and all others who value
the computational modeling and its power.*

Contents

Preface

Biology is becoming more and more of a quantitative science, some even say that it is at a stage similar to physics pre-Newton [16]. It is waiting for break-throughs not only in terms of biological discoveries but also in terms of new methods that will catalyse them, similar to Newton's mechanics being catalysed by the development of calculus.

At the same time, experiments using computer simulations have become very accessible and in some cases even preferable to biological experiments. The computational resources today are fairly easily available and can be used to test various hypotheses before diving into more complicated or expensive biological testing procedures.

These two trends are steadily converging and attract considerable attention in both the biomedical and the computational fields. How did we find ourselves in the middle of it?

Both of us are trained mathematicians. We have studied numerical analysis, optimisation and mathematical modeling. Our paths had briefly crossed at the Comenius University in Bratislava, Slovakia, where we both got our master's degrees in Mathematics but then led us on to separate trails. Ivan to Ghent University, Belgium and Fachhochschule St. Poelten, Austria and Iveta to New Jersey Institute of Technology, Newark, USA. During this time, we both somehow intuitively navigated towards more applied topics and when we met again at University of Žilina it was on a project to model red blood cells in microfluidic devices.

Looking back, the beginnings of the project seem more like a random walk than a steady progress towards a good model. Two steps forward, one step back. And then another to a dead-end sidetrack. Yes, research is like that but talking together some time later we both agreed that it could have been easier. Had we known some more basics about membrane biomechanics and about building cell models, we could have saved ourselves quite a bit of time and frustration.

With that hope we are writing this book. We would like to help young researchers entering this promising field and professionals who could use blood cell models in their applied work get oriented and started. We focus on cell mechanics and specifically red blood cell mechanics, even though we briefly touch upon other types of blood cells and circulating tumor cells. Computational blood cell models are useful in many applications such as diagnostics of diseases using various lab-on-a-chip concepts, monitoring of response to treatment and also in primary research of blood flow and its properties.

Red blood cells perform several biological functions and their abilities directly depend on their shape and structural stiffness. The cells respond to external mechanical stimuli and interact with their surroundings by changing their shapes or mechanical properties, which may even lead to their damage under extreme conditions. Cell models have to account for complex processes that happen at varied length scales - from molecular to microscale, at which the cells live, and still conform to the macro behavior of cell flow. That is not an easy task and we would like if this book could help in tackling it.

Some things this book is not. It is not a universal book on building models in general. While certainly invaluable, that kind of book would be extremely difficult to write and quite difficult to use once one wants to build a specific model, e.g. a model of a cell. We try to point out some general principles of building good models, but more often than not, the principles we mention apply specifically to cell models. Also this book is not an exhaustive treatment of all computational cell models out there. We try to set things into context and perspective by giving the reader some background, but our main focus is to help a modeler new to the field of blood cell modeling overcome initial hurdles and distill what is essential. We do not cover biological or chemical processes inside the cell, but rather remain on the whole cell scale.

We hope that the book will help the readers see models as bridges between different levels of understanding and that it will inspire new work in the exciting and very promising field of cell modeling.

Ivan Cimrák and Iveta Jančigová
Žilina, Slovakia

Acknowledgements

We are very grateful to our colleagues and PhD students at University of Žilina who have read the first drafts of this book, commented on them, criticised and made us do better: Katarína Bachratá, Kristína Kovalčíková, Alžbeta Bohiníková, Mariana Ondrušová, Monika Smiešková, Martin Slavík and Hynek Bachratý.

We also want to thank two anonymous reviewers who have offered many valuable suggestions, which helped us significantly improve the book.

Some of the mentioned work has been done with colleagues Renáta Tóthová and Martin Bušík while they were at University of Žilina and with Markus Gusenbauer and Giulia Mazza from Danube University Krems.

A number of people have read parts of the book and offered their constructive perspectives: Ondrej Šuch, Katarína Borovičková, Mirka Cimráková, Daniel Ševčovič, Ľubomír Baňas, Aleksey Belyaev and Denisa Maceková.

We thank Sofie Caroline De Bruyne for design of the cover.

Thanks also to our department and faculty who have supported our work and to people at the Institute of Computational Physics in Stuttgart, who take care of the open-source ESPResSo project and its contributors like us.

Finally, thanks to our editors Safraz Khan, Callum Fraser and Linda Leggio for their patience and guidance in getting this book from our heads into reality.

Symbols and Abbreviations

A, B, C, D, X_i	points in space
x, y, z	axes in Cartesian coordinate system
t	time variable
$\theta, \phi, \alpha, \beta$	angles
$\mathbf{a}, \mathbf{r}_i, \mathbf{t}_A$	vectors
$\mathbf{n}, \mathbf{n}_{ABC}$	normal vectors, associated to plane given by ABC
$\mathbf{A}, \mathbf{B}, \mathbf{C}, \mathbf{D}, \mathbf{X}_i$	position vectors of points in space
$\mathbf{F}, \mathbf{F}_i, \mathbf{F}_s$	force vectors
$\mathbf{T}$	torque vectors
$\mathbf{a} = [a_x, a_y, a_z]$	vector $\mathbf{a}$ and its components
$|\mathbf{a}|$	length or magnitude of vector $\mathbf{a}$
$\mathbf{A} \times \mathbf{B}$	cross-product of two vectors
$(\mathbf{a}, \mathbf{b})$	dot product of vectors $\mathbf{a}$ and $\mathbf{b}$
$\frac{df(t)}{dt}, \frac{df}{dt}$	derivative of f with respect to t
J	deformation matrix
S, S_0	surface area
V, V_0	volume
n, n_i, n_{cell}	number of objects or items
Δx	spatial discretisation step
Δt	temporal discretisation step
k_s	elastic coefficient for stretching
k_b	elastic coefficient for bending
k_{al}	elastic coefficient for local area
k_{ag}	elastic coefficient for global area
k_v	elastic coefficient for volume
k_{visc}	elastic coefficient for viscosity
μ	dynamic viscosity of the fluid
ρ	density of the fluid
$\dot{\gamma}$	shear rate
τ, τ_{xy}	shear stress
σ_{xx}	normal stress
ϵ, ϵ_{xy}	strain, shear strain
P	pressure
Q	volumetric flow rate

ν	Poisson's ratio
Y	Young's modulus
μ_0	shear modulus
K	area compression/expansion modulus
k_c	bending modulus
η_m	viscosity modulus
k_V	osmotic modulus
t_c	cell relaxation time
Re	Reynolds number
Ca	capillary number
Ma	lattice Mach number
c_s	lattice speed of sound
ξ, ξ_{ref}	friction parameter for fluid-structure coupling
$\mathcal{W}$	virial of the system of particles
P_a	capture rate
k_B	Boltzmann constant

ACDG	**A**veraged **C**umulative **D**eviation of **G**lobal area
BC	**B**oundary **C**onditions
BDI	**B**lood **D**amage **I**ndex
CDG	**C**umulative **D**eviation of **G**lobal area
CDI	**C**ell **D**amage **I**ndex
CpR	**C**ollision **p**er **R**ow
CTC	**C**irculating **T**umor **C**ell
D3Q19	**D**imensions **3** velocities **19**, a specific implementation of the lattice-Boltzmann method
DI	**D**eformation **I**ndex
DPD	**D**issipative **P**article **D**ynamics
ESPResSo	**E**xtensible **S**imulation **P**ackage for **Res**earch on **So**ft Matter, scientific software package
FENE	**F**inite **E**xtensible **N**on-linear **E**lastic
GEDI	**G**eometrically **E**nhanced **D**ifferential **I**mmunocapture
GUI	**G**raphical **U**ser **I**nterface
Ht	**H**ematocrit
IB-DC	**I**mmersed **B**oundary - **D**issipative **C**oupling
IBM	**I**mmersed **B**oundary **M**ethod
LBM	**L**attice-**B**oltzmann **M**ethod
LOC	**L**ab-**O**n-a-**C**hip
MPI	**M**essage **P**assing **I**nterface
ParaView	**Para**llel **V**isualisation application
PDMS	**P**oly-**D**i-**M**ethyl-**S**iloxane
PER	**P**assive **E**lastic **R**igidity
POA	**P**eriodic **O**bstacle **A**rray
POC	**P**oint-**O**f-**C**are
RBC	**R**ed **B**lood **C**ell

SPH	**S**moothed **P**article **H**ydrodynamics
VAD	**V**entricular **A**ssist **D**evice
WBC	**W**hite **B**lood **C**ell
WLC	**W**orm-**L**ike **C**hain

Chapter 1

Introduction

1.1   Computational modeling as a tool for understanding

The question *Why modeling?* has already been answered many times and we suspect that by answering it again here, we are preaching to the converted. But instead of brushing it aside by stating that the importance of computational modeling is self-evident, we sketch a few examples here. We do that in the hopes that these examples will also spark the *self-evidence idea* for those who have not been exposed to computational modeling at all and are now wondering.

The first example is from the US National Institute of Biomedical Imaging and Bioengineering [143]. Suppose we want to bake a cake. With a dozen ingredients, there are many possibilities in how to combine them. Having a computer model of baking the cake, we could run multiple simulations with different amounts of ingredients to see how the cake turns out.

With such a computer model, it is even possible to try how skipping one, two or even more ingredients would affect the taste or the structure of the cake. For one ingredient, there are 20 possibilities and in principle, this could also be done by baking 20 cakes. Almost no effect when skipping raisins. Not including flour brings on a small disaster. Leaving out two ingredients results in 190 new cakes, without three ingredients we have 1140 cakes and skipping four ingredients brings us to 4845 possibilities. Imagine baking 4845 different cakes. Compared to that, running 4845 simulations is easy. This example may not be too convincing, because we do not get to taste the computational cake with our tongues.

So let us now consider a thermo-mechanical model of a skyscraper. Using such a model, we can shake the skyscraper (effectively modeling an earthquake and we do not have to try just one, but many earthquakes of different strengths), let the skyscraper burn (modeling spreading of fire from specific locations) or let the skyscraper age (modeling the durability of the materials and the building itself).

These examples illustrate maybe the most significant advantage of computational modeling: the ability to answer the *What if?* questions about complex real systems that cannot be answered in reality. After all, no one would ever build a hundred skyscrapers to see what design gives the best protection against earthquakes, right?

As our book title says, we work (mostly) with models of red blood cells. These cells lead an active and tough life. They return to the heart about once every minute of their 100-120 day lifespan. Each time they visit the spleen, they pass a fitness test squeezing through a narrow opening. They are subject to various stresses and deformations while bringing oxygen to all our other cells and removing the carbon dioxide.

Models of these cells need to reflect their capabilities reasonably well and to achieve that, several parameters have to be included and carefully calibrated. Then we can vary the situations, to which we expose the modeled cells and investigate the effects both from theoretical and applicational points of view.

Performing simulation studies and examining responses to changes in parameters - this is called sensitivity analysis - are just some of the possible uses of good models. In addition to them, computational models let us test hypotheses, suggest and interpret experiments, uncover causation, bring new insights and inspire future work - also for experimentalists - and more.

Who can benefit from this book?
We have already indicated the target group of readers for this book in the Preface. There we have also mentioned reasons that motivated us for writing this book. One of them is *to make the life of young researchers easier*. *Young* is meant as *new in the cell modeling business*. Indeed, we think this book could be helpful for advanced master students, doctoral students, as well as established researchers starting their journey in cell modeling. Some of you may have previous experience with modeling in other areas and of course, if you do, you will have a slight advantage over the modeling newcomers, but it is not expected at this point.

If you have some basic background specifically in cell modeling, you may benefit from the book as well. Besides the general sections with ideas valid for any modeling, we often relate the presented concepts to other approaches and highlight differences or similarities.

1.2   Compass over map

Overall, we have written this book in a context we call *compass over map*. We want to give the reader a compass and explain how to use it, instead of giving him or her a detailed map with a precisely indicated route from point A to point B. We believe this is much more useful once they want to go to point C, especially in situations, when it is unclear, what the *correct* route is. The correctness of the route depends on the criteria the modeler sets in advance. Therefore, rather than explain how everything is, we try to describe how to look for a direction, how to find it and how to get to the desired models.

In this book, we build computational models step by step. We expect these models to give us correct answers to questions about reality. The models do not have to correspond to reality in all aspects, only to such extent that they give us answers to the questions of interest.

For us, a red blood cell is *the object* that we always have in mind. So, in this book, we identify the shape and structure of this object. We determine the mechanical properties of the materials, of which this object consists. We describe the behavior of the object using the fundamental laws of physics and we implement them into a numerical model.

In order to test the model, we create a code that is capable of simulating the cell behavior. To link the real cells to our model cells, we calibrate the model parameters using experimental measurements of basic cell manipulation. Then we validate the computational model against more complex physiological experiments. And when needed, we return to some of the previous points. While the focus is on red blood cells, the steps are general enough that other types of cells could in principle be considered.

Having done all this, we can finally approach those *What if?* questions and use the validated model to predict outcomes of other experiments and to formulate hypotheses.

The *compass over map* approach should also urge the readers and modelers to think about models, whether those we present here or some others, with constructive doubts and to have some reality-check questions simmering on the back burner. For example: *What do you know about the system post-model, that you did not know pre-model?* This type of questioning keeps you grounded whether the model is actually useful. Another useful question that should have a reasonable answer is: *Once you have a model and you have indicated all the data your model does explain, what data does it not explain?*

A model is always a simplification of reality and as such, it necessarily omits some properties or features. We need to be aware of that. (We will point out examples like this later in the book.) And of course, what about apparent flaws? *Be sensitive and keep track of them.* Keep an eye out for how they can be explained. Double check. Many of them lead to the discovery of model flaws. Triple check. If they are still there, consider whether the theory needs to be changed to fit them.

The thing is though that modeling is not a spectator sport. It requires countless hours of practice, a lot of sweat and, in our case, literally also blood. (No worries, the blood will only be inside your computer.) That is one of the reasons why we accompany the text with simulation scripts - snippets in text and full scripts online - that can be used alongside the book to support the presented concepts. A few of them illustrate some of the mistakes that we have made. They use the Object-in-fluid package that we developed and included in ESPResSo - open-source scientific software for simulations of soft matter [31, 32]. We believe the scripts are an essential and inseparable part of this work.

The Achilles heel of books with code

Books about coding and more general, books containing snippets of code of any particular language or software, have one big disadvantage: As soon as the language or software evolves, the book becomes in some sense outdated. The commands presented in such a book may no longer be available in the next versions of that software. We face the same problem: ESPResSo with its Object-in-fluid module is a live project, it evolves, grows and adapts to new ideas.

The snippets presented in this book are linked to its 4.0 release. So even at a later date, with this version of ESPResSo, they should work.

We believe that this book will remain timely even if some commands have different forms in the future. The concepts stay the same and the current syntax may be found in the up-to-date documentation online.

We are also using these supplementary materials to guide our own students along. We encourage them to contemplate a question before presenting an answer to it. From our experience, giving people results before the problem bothers them enough does not make for a proper understanding. That is the reason why some topics are not presented in the text just once, in their final form, but rather we present them first in a more naïve manner and then return to them once the consequences are evident and need to be addressed.

1.3   How to read this book

Throughout the book, the grey boxes such as the one in the previous section add some commentary to the topic being discussed, something like a handwritten thought on the margin. We also use these grey boxes when we want to wrap up an idea, summarise certain terminology and findings or point out connections between the presented topics.

Sometimes, we intentionally do not mention all the details or all the consequences of the discussed issue. We leave space for the reader to raise some questions about the missing information. At the same time, we do not want them to get lost. Therefore, we collect the questions about potential caveats of what was just said and things to try in order to help understanding. At certain places in the text, we pose these questions and suggestions as *Things to ponder*.

Things to ponder
How can I get the most out of this book? How should I read it?

While the book certainly can be read in a linear fashion, we understand that different readers expect different insights and several alternative paths through the book are possible. Here we offer a brief description of each chapter to let the reader decide.

Chapter 2 *Illustrative simulation example* describes an introductory simulation that presents a computer script. It explains some of the possibilities and available features step by step. If you are interested mainly in building a model or if you have previous experience with cell modeling, this chapter may be skipped. It is primarily meant for readers not familiar with these topics to illustrate basic outcomes and to make it a bit clearer what we are trying to achieve. An alternative to reading this chapter is watching a video at www.compbloodcell.eu.

Chapter 3 *Cell model* contains the modeling core of the book. Here, we establish the cell model (Sections 3.2, 3.3), first with some hidden flaws but then revisited (Section 3.4) and improved. The modeling part is complemented with Section 3.5, which discusses the fluid solver and Section 3.6, which addresses the cell-cell interactions. The cell model is then discussed within the context of other approaches in Section 3.7.

To link the biological reality with the developed model, in Chapter 4 *Model vs. bioreality* we first review and derive theoretical foundations (Section 4.2) and then we use the theory as a starting point for direct comparison of model and real-world experiments with cells in Section 4.3. Data from experiments need to be approached carefully and in Section 4.4 we point out several issues that should be considered.

After this chapter, the model is ready for practical use, but before we actually use it, in Chapter 5 *Practical issues* we point out some issues that may arise. These include strategies for seeding of dense simulations or suitable discretisations.

In Chapter 6 *Applications*, we describe some - with absolutely no intention of being exhaustive - applications of the presented model. We show how this model may be used for computing capture rates of circulating tumor cells in microfluidic devices (Section 6.4) or for evaluating collision rates during deterministic lateral displacement in periodic obstacle arrays (Section 6.5). The knowledge of individual cell deformation during the passage of the device may be used for evaluation of the blood damage index (Section 6.6) and for design optimisation of ventricular assist devices (Section 6.7). The user-friendly open-source approach in computer implementation of the model has also led to its use for optimisation of micro-roughness of channel surfaces (Section 6.8).

The model, or more precisely, the force-based approach to cell modeling, is flexible enough that several other biological phenomena, such as cell adhesion, inclusion of a cell's inner structure or modeling of stiff cells can be tried. These ideas are explored in Chapter 7 *Ideas for extension*.

Chapter 8 does not contain either *Conclusions* or *Summary*. It is called *Dreaming up the future* and in it we discuss, where the modeling may lead some time in the future. While writing this chapter, we have unleashed our imagination a little bit and we have replaced the *sci-entific* context with a *sci-fiction* context.

In order not to clutter the text and let the core ideas sufficiently stand out in the main text, we have collected the more tedious calculations, derivations and specific details that are needed for completeness in the Appendices.

Chapter 2

Illustrative simulation example

2.1 Why simulation before modeling?

The title of this book promises cell models. And here we are, at the beginning, and instead of diving directly into modeling, we are going to take a look at a simulation first. We do that because we want to create images in your mind for later. Once we start talking about elasticity, we want you to already have seen an elastic cell deform. Once we talk about validation of the model and correspondence to reality, we want you to have some idea, what kind of inputs such a simulation needs and what kind of outputs it can provide.

The second reason is that the example in this chapter is simplified and self-contained, but with the help of the code snippets in the following chapters, it can be extended and adapted for performing various more accurate and more sophisticated simulation experiments with the cell. We want you to have this opportunity from the beginning and encourage you to give it a try.

Later, we also point out a few things that do not work or do not work well. It is therefore useful, to have something that works at the beginning, to have something to compare to. After all, as we were writing this book, the working title of this chapter has been *A simple simulation that works*.

It is certainly not required to work through this particular simulation now, especially if you have previous experience with cell modeling or prefer to start with model building and returning here later. As supplementary material, we have also prepared a short video that shows these steps and visualises the results. It is available at www.compbloodcell.eu.

2.2 Basic setup

The simulation script we are going to look at is written in Python language. While it is useful to have some background in Python, we will go over the script step by step so that those who do not speak Python (yet) will also start to understand the basic vocabulary and phrases.

This is a script that creates a red blood cell and lets it flow in fluid. To try it out yourself, you need to have a machine with ESPResSo 4.0 installed. Details on how to do that can be found in the ESPResSo user guides [95, 100].

The simulation script and two input files are also available at the second website. It is possible that by the time you are reading this text, a newer version of ESPResSo or of the Object-in-fluid module is available. The 4.0 release should still work as described here, while for a later version, it is possible that the syntax may have evolved a little bit. The online documentation available at [100] should explain all about the current version.

ESPResSo

Extensible **S**imulation **P**ackage for **Res**earch on **So**ft Matter is a modular parallel engine for soft matter simulations [7]. While primarily aimed at molecular dynamics, it can also efficiently simulate microscale elastic objects. The computational engine does not run from a graphical user interface (GUI), visualise simulations or plot output data, but it has a Python scripting interface that can be used for setting up the simulations, data post-processing, plotting and saving output for later visualisation. We have implemented an Object-in-fluid module [31] that can be used for simulations of closed elastic objects.

The computational engine of ESPResSo is written in C++. You might wonder why there is the scripting interface to control the simulation at all. Why not just have a graphical application built on top of the computational core, where you select some domain, number of cells, maybe some of their properties and then run it by clicking a button? While certainly easier, this approach would be very limiting. What if you want to measure some characteristics of your cells that are not available in the default application? What if you want to run a completely different geometry or setup not offered in the application menu? The scripting interface gives you infinitely more freedom than a GUI.

Besides the standard Python commands and funcionality, the scripting interface uses basic building blocks - cells, fluid, boundaries, etc. - and lets you combine and examine them as you want. Moreover, after a short introduction, Python is a very friendly beast. Come, take a look.

In the first few lines, the script includes several imports related to the red blood cell model and fluid - some of those building blocks that we have mentioned.

```
1   import espressomd
2   import object_in_fluid as oif
3   from espressomd import lb
4   import numpy as np
5
6   system = espressomd.System(box_l=[22.0, 14.0, 14.0])
7   system.time_step = 0.1
8   system.cell_system.skin = 0.2
9
10  # creating the template for RBCs
11  type = oif.OifCellType(nodes_file="input/rbc374nodes.dat", \
12  triangles_file="input/rbc374triangles.dat", system=system, \
13  ks=0.02, kb=0.016, kal=0.02, kag=0.9, kv=0.5, resize=[2.0, 2.0, 2.0])
14
15  # creating the RBCs
16  cell = oif.OifCell(cell_type=type, particle_type=0, \
17  origin=[5.0, 5.0, 3.0])
18  cell.output_vtk_pos_folded(file_name="output/sim1/cell_0.vtk")
19
20  # fluid
21  lbf = espressomd.lb.LBFluid(agrid=1, dens=1.0, visc=1.5, \
22  tau=system.time_step, fric=1.5, ext_force=[0.002, 0.0, 0.0])
23  system.actors.add(lbf)
24
25  # main integration loop
26  maxCycle = 100
27  for i in range(1, maxCycle):
28          system.integrator.run(steps=500)
29          cell.output_vtk_pos_folded(file_name="output/sim1/cell_" \
30          + str(i) + ".vtk")
31          print "time: ", str(i*system.time_step*500)
32  print "Simulation completed."
```

In lines 6-8, we set up an ESPResSo system and its most important parameters.

```
6   system = espressomd.System(box_l=[22.0, 14.0, 14.0])
7   system.time_step = 0.1
8   system.cell_system.skin = 0.2
```

The skin depth tunes the system's performance. The computed results will be the same, no matter what value of skin is chosen, however, the time needed for simulation can differ quite significantly. We discuss *skin* in more detail in Section 5.5 within a bullet list concerning cell-cell interactions.

The attribute box_l represents the dimensions of the 3D simulation box. You might wonder what the units are. We talk about these in Appendix F.1, but for now, you can think of them as micrometers.

The attribute `time_step` stores the time step that will be used in the simulation, for the purposes here, in microseconds. ESPResSo allows separate specification of time step for the particles and for the fluid. This is useful when one also takes into account thermal fluctuations of the membrane, i.e. processes on the molecular level, which is much finer scale than we work at. For us, both of these time steps will be identical.

```
11    type = oif.OifCellType(nodes_file="input/rbc374nodes.dat", \
12    triangles_file="input/rbc374triangles.dat", system=system, \
13    ks=0.02, kb=0.016, kal=0.02, kag=0.9, kv=0.5, resize=[2.0, 2.0, 2.0])
```

We do not create elastic objects directly but rather each one has to correspond to a template, `type`, that has been created first. The advantage of this approach is clear when creating many objects of the same type that only differ by, e.g. position or rotation, because in such case it significantly speeds up the creation of objects that are just copies of the same template.

The three mandatory parameters are `nodes-file` and `triangles-file` that specify input data files with the desired triangulation and `system` that specifies the ESPResSo system. More on triangulation can be found in Chapter 3. While the lengths of triangulation edges vary during the simulation, the connectivity of the mesh nodes never changes. This script assumes that the two necessary files are located inside an `input` directory that resides in the same folder as the simulation script.

Files for this simulation example
Basic triangulation meshes can be downloaded from our website together with the Object-in-fluid documentation, which also explains the format and how to make custom triangulation meshes should you need them.

All other arguments are optional. Argument `resize` allows resizing in the x, y, z directions with respect to unit size of the object, so in this case, the cell radius will be 2. Arguments `ks`, `kb`, `kal`, `kag` and `kv` specify the elastic properties: stretching, bending, local area conservation, global area conservation and volume conservation, respectively. More about these elastic moduli can be found in Chapter 3 and more details on calibration and how to obtain the proper values in Section 4.3.1.

The keywords can come in any order. The backslash allows the long command to continue over multiple lines.

```
16    cell = oif.OifCell(cell_type=type, particle_type=0, \
17    origin=[5.0, 5.0, 3.0])
18    cell.output_vtk_pos_folded(file_name="output/sim1/cell_0.vtk")
```

Next, an actual object is created and its initial position is saved to a *.vtk* file (the directory output/sim1 needs to exist before the script is run). Each object has to have a unique ID, specified using the keyword particle_type. The IDs have to start at 0 and increase consecutively. The other two mandatory parameters are cell_type and origin. The parameter cell_type specifies which previously defined cell type will be used for this object. The parameter origin gives the placement of the object's center in the simulation box.

```
21   lbf = espressomd.lb.LBFluid(agrid=1, dens=1.0, visc=1.5, \
22   tau=system.time_step, fric=1.5, ext_force=[0.002, 0.0, 0.0])
23   system.actors.add(lbf)
```

This part of the script specifies the fluid that will get the system moving. Here agrid $= \Delta x$ is the spatial discretisation step, tau is the time step that will be the same as the time step for particles and kinematic viscosity visc and density dens of the fluid are physical parameters scaled to lattice units (as already mentioned, more information on units can be found in Appendix F.1). Parameter fric enters the fluid-object interaction and has to be set carefully (Section 3.5). Finally, ext_force sets the force-per-unit-volume vector that drives the fluid. It is similar to pressure difference at the beginning and end of a simulated chamber - the larger it is, the faster flow it induces. Another option to add momentum to fluid is by specifying the velocity on the boundaries (more details in the Object-in-fluid user guide).

And finally, the heart of this script is the integration loop at the end:

```
26   maxCycle = 100
27   for i in range(1, maxCycle):
28          system.integrator.run(steps=500)
29          cell.OutputVtkPosFolded(filename="output/sim1/cell_" \
30          + str(i) + ".vtk")
31          print "time: ", str(i*system.time_step*500)
32   print "Simulation completed."
```

This simulation runs for 100 cycles. In each cycle, 500 integration steps are performed and output is saved into files output/sim1/cell_i.vtk. Note that the file names differ only by the number before the .vtk extension stored in variable i. This variable changes due to the for loop and this will allow us to animate the output in the visualisation software. str changes the type of i from integer to string, so that it can be used in the filename. The strings can be joined together by the + sign. Also, in each pass of the loop, the simulation time is printed in the terminal window and when the integration is complete, we should get a message about it.

So now that we know what is in the script, we can run it in a terminal window using the command line:

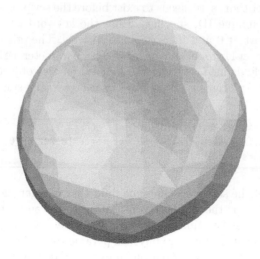

FIGURE 2.1: Screenshot from the simulation, using visualisation software ParaView [90].

```
path_to_executable/./pypresso script.py
```

Here `script.py` is the name of the script we just went over. This command assumes that we are currently in the same directory as the script. Once the command is executed, notifications about the integration steps appear in the terminal window:

```
time:   0.1
time:   0.2
time:   0.3
```

If everything went well, there should be plenty of .vtk files in the directory `output/sim1`. Let us take a look at what we have there. For visualisation, we suggest the freely available software ParaView [90]. All .vtk files can be loaded at the same time as a sequence using the Open icon. Then we can run an animation using the play button in the center of the top toolbar. The visualised cell should look similar to Figure 2.1.

Things to ponder
Woo-hoo. Now what?

2.3 Adding more complexity

The simulation that we just performed was indeed quite simple. Not too many characters, not much of a plot. So let us add a few things: boundaries, obstacles, another cell or two and see what else is needed as a consequence. First, we start with creating the output directory sim2 and modifying the output lines accordingly.

To add another cell, we can use either the same or different cellType. Here, we are using the same one:

```
cell1 = OifCell(cell_type=type, particle_type=1, origin=[5.0, 5.0, 7.0], \
rotate=[0.0, pi/2, 0.0], particle_mass=0.5)
cell1.output_vtk_pos_folded(file_name="output/sim2/cell1_0.vtk")
```

This cell has a different particle_type than the first cell, so that we can differentiate between the two types of particles later. The two optional parameters are rotate and particle_mass. Parameter rotate takes three arguments - angles in radians - that determine how much the object is rotated around the x, y, z axes. The keyword particle_mass takes one value and this mass is assigned to each surface node of the object.

Two types of boundaries are specified next: four walls of the chamber (top, bottom, front and back) and three cylindrical obstacles. We do not need the remaining two walls, because the fluid flowing in positive x direction (due to the applied external force) flows from the left to the right.

For each obstacle or boundary, we define its shape:

```
tmp_shape = shapes.Rhomboid(corner=[0.0, 0.0, 0.0], a=[boxX, 0.0, 0.0], \
b=[0.0, boxY, 0.0], c=[0.0, 0.0, 1.0], direction=1)
```

Note that the rhomboid wall or obstacle is defined by its corner and then three vectors a,b,c that go from the corner to the three neighboring corners, as depicted in Figure 2.2. The order of the vectors is important and should follow the right-hand rule, so that the inside/outside is properly defined. The cylinder obstacle is defined by its center, axis, length and radius:

```
tmp_shape = shapes.Cylinder(center=[11.0, 2.0, 7.0], \
axis=[0.0, 0.0, 1.0], length=14.0, radius=2.0, direction=1)
```

For both types of obstacles, direction specifies whether the simulated region is outside the boundary (direction= 1) or inside it (direction= −1).

Once we have the shape, we define the fluid boundary:

```
system.lbboundaries.add(lbboundaries.LBBoundary(shape=tmp_shape))
```

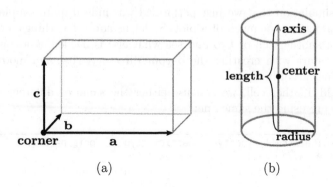

(a)　　　　　　　　　　　　　　(b)

FIGURE 2.2: Two of the boundary types: (a) Rhomboid defined by its corner and three vectors **a**, **b**, **c**. (b) Cylinder defined by its center, radius, length and axis.

We also define a boundary for particles representing the cell surface using the same shape. One may wonder why it is necessary to define separate boundaries for the fluid and for particles forming the cell boundary. This is caused by using two different solvers, one for the fluid and one for the particles. Let us skip the details for now, they can be found in Section 3.1.4.

Note the keyword `particle_type` in this definition. It denotes similar type as `particle_type` that was defined for particles and will be used later for interactions:

```
system.constraints.add(shape=tmp_shape, particle_type=10, penetrable=0)
```

And we output the boundary for later visualisations:

```
oif.output_vtk_rhomboid(rhom_shape=tmp_shape, \
out_file="output/sim2/wallBottom.vtk")
```

The same steps are repeated for all boundaries, so they can be performed in a cycle.

A visual check before running a simulation
It is a good idea to output and visualise the boundaries and objects just prior to running the actual simulation. This is the reason why we have also saved the cells with the index 0 before the integration loop. We

can visualise them together with the boundaries to make sure that the geometry is correct and no objects intersect with any boundaries.

Now we use the `particle_type` of the boundaries (unlike the cells, all boundaries can have the same type) and define the cell-wall interactions:

```
system.non_bonded_inter[0,10].soft_sphere.set_params( \
a = 0.0001, n = 1.2, cutoff = 0.1, offset = 0.0)
system.non_bonded_inter[1,10].soft_sphere.set_params( \
a = 0.0001, n = 1.2, cutoff = 0.1, offset = 0.0)
```

These interactions are *pointwise*, e.g. each particle of type 0 (that means all mesh points of `cell`) will have a repulsive soft-sphere interaction with all boundaries of type 10 (here all boundaries) once it gets closer than `cutoff`. Also, all particles of type 1 (mesh points of `cell1`) will have the same repulsive interaction with the boundaries. The parameters `a` and `n` adjust how strong the interaction is and `offset` is zero for our purposes. We provide guidelines on how to set proper values in Appendix F.4.

Since we now have two cells, we can and should also set up the cell-cell interactions so that they *know* about each other:

```
system.non_bonded_inter[0,1].membrane_collision.set_params(\
a = 0.0001, n = 1.2, cutoff = 0.1, offset = 0.0)
```

These interactions also act *pointwise* like the cell-wall interactions, e.g. each particle of type 0 (all mesh points of `cell`) has a repulsive membrane collision interaction with each particle of type 1 (all mesh points of `cell1`) once the pair gets closer than `cutoff`. For this interaction to work, we also need to add the parameter `normal=True` when creating the `cellType`. This will ensure that the cells know the outward direction of their membrane and can properly interact with each other. More details on the ideas behind these interactions can be found in Section 3.6.

Here is the complete script:

```
1   import espressomd
2   import object_in_fluid as oif
3   from espressomd import lb
4   from espressomd import lbboundaries
5   from espressomd import shapes
6   from espressomd import interactions
7   import numpy as np
8
9   boxX = 22.0
10  boxY = 14.0
11  boxZ = 14.0
```

```
12   system = espressomd.System(box_l=[boxX, boxY, boxZ])
13   system.cell_system.skin = 0.2
14   system.time_step = 0.1
15
16   # creating the template for RBCs
17   type = oif.OifCellType(nodes_file="input/rbc374nodes.dat", \
18   triangles_file="input/rbc374triangles.dat", check_orientation=False, \
19   system=system, ks=0.02, kb=0.016, kal=0.02, kag=0.9, kv=0.5, \
20   resize=[2.0, 2.0, 2.0], normal=True)
21
22   # creating the RBCs
23   cell = oif.OifCell(cell_type=type, particle_type=0, \
24   origin=[5.0, 5.0, 3.0])
25   cell1 = oif.OifCell(cell_type=type, particle_type=1, \
26   origin=[5.0, 5.0, 7.0], rotate=[0.0, np.pi/2, 0.0], particle_mass=0.5)
27
28   print "Cells created."
29
30   # fluid
31   lbf = espressomd.lb.LBFluid(agrid=1, dens=1.0, visc=1.5, \
32   tau=system.time_step, fric=1.5, ext_force=[0.002, 0.0, 0.0])
33   system.actors.add(lbf)
34
35   boundaries = []
36
37   # bottom of the channel
38   tmp_shape = shapes.Rhomboid(corner=[0.0, 0.0, 0.0], \
39   a=[boxX, 0.0, 0.0], b=[0.0, boxY, 0.0], c=[0.0, 0.0, 1.0], direction=1)
40   boundaries.append(tmp_shape)
41   oif.output_vtk_rhomboid(rhom_shape=tmp_shape, \
42   out_file="output/sim2/wallBottom.vtk")
43
44   # top of the channel
45   tmp_shape = shapes.Rhomboid(corner=[0.0, 0.0, boxZ-1], \
46   a=[boxX, 0.0, 0.0], b=[0.0, boxY, 0.0], c=[0.0, 0.0, 1.0], direction=1)
47   boundaries.append(tmp_shape)
48   oif.output_vtk_rhomboid(rhom_shape=tmp_shape, \
49   out_file="output/sim2/wallTop.vtk")
50
51   # front wall of the channel
52   tmp_shape = shapes.Rhomboid(corner=[0.0, 0.0, 0.0], \
53   a=[boxX, 0.0, 0.0], b=[0.0, 1.0, 0.0], c=[0.0, 0.0, boxZ], direction=1)
54   boundaries.append(tmp_shape)
55   oif.output_vtk_rhomboid(rhom_shape=tmp_shape, \
56   out_file="output/sim2/wallFront.vtk")
57
58   # back wall of the channel
59   tmp_shape = shapes.Rhomboid(corner=[0.0, boxY-1.0, 0.0], \
60   a=[boxX, 0.0, 0.0], b=[0.0, 1.0, 0.0], c=[0.0, 0.0, boxZ], direction=1)
```

```
61    boundaries.append(tmp_shape)
62    oif.output_vtk_rhomboid(rhom_shape=tmp_shape, \
63    out_file="output/sim2/wallBack.vtk")
64
65    # obstacle - cylinder A
66    tmp_shape = shapes.Cylinder(center=[11.0, 2.0, 7.0], \
67    axis=[0.0, 0.0, 1.0], length=14.0, radius=2.0, direction=1)
68    boundaries.append(tmp_shape)
69    oif.output_vtk_cylinder(cyl_shape=tmp_shape, n=20, \
70    out_file="output/sim2/cylinderA.vtk")
71
72    # obstacle - cylinder B
73    tmp_shape = shapes.Cylinder(center=[16.0, 8.0, 7.0], \
74    axis=[0.0, 0.0, 1.0], length=14.0, radius=2.0, direction=1)
75    boundaries.append(tmp_shape)
76    oif.output_vtk_cylinder(cyl_shape=tmp_shape, n=20, \
77    out_file="output/sim2/cylinderB.vtk")
78
79    # obstacle - cylinder C
80    tmp_shape = shapes.Cylinder(center=[11.0, 12.0, 7.0], \
81    axis=[0.0, 0.0, 1.0], length=14.0, radius=2.0, direction=1)
82    boundaries.append(tmp_shape)
83    oif.output_vtk_cylinder(cyl_shape=tmp_shape, n=20, \
84    out_file="output/sim2/cylinderC.vtk")
85
86    for boundary in boundaries:
87        system.lbboundaries.add(lbboundaries.LBBoundary(shape=boundary))
88        system.constraints.add(shape=boundary, particle_type=10, \
89        penetrable=0)
90
91    print "Boundaries created."
92
93    # cell-wall interactions
94    system.non_bonded_inter[0, 10].soft_sphere.set_params(a=0.0001, \
95    n=1.2, cutoff=0.1, offset=0.0)
96    system.non_bonded_inter[1, 10].soft_sphere.set_params(a=0.0001, \
97    n=1.2, cutoff=0.1, offset=0.0)
98
99    # cell-cell interactions
100   system.non_bonded_inter[0, 1].membrane_collision.set_params(\
101   a=0.0001, n=1.2, cutoff=0.1, offset=0.0)
102
103   print "Interactions created."
104
105   maxCycle = 100
106   # main integration loop
107   cell.output_vtk_pos_folded(file_name="output/sim2/cell_0.vtk")
108   cell1.output_vtk_pos_folded(file_name="output/sim2/cell1_0.vtk")
109   for i in range(1, maxCycle):
```

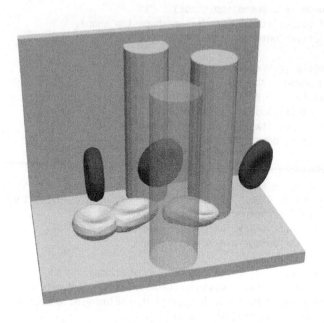

FIGURE 2.3: An overlay of three screenshots from a simulation with two cells (dark and light) using visualisation software ParaView [90]. The front and top walls are not shown. The column in front has lowered opacity, so that we also see the cells passing behind it.

```
110     system.integrator.run(steps=500)
111     cell.output_vtk_pos_folded(file_name="output/sim2/cell_"\
112     + str(i) + ".vtk")
113     cell1.output_vtk_pos_folded(file_name="output/sim2/cell1_"\
114     + str(i) + ".vtk")
115     print "time: ", str(i*system.time_step*500)
116  print "Simulation completed."
117
```

After running the simulation, the visualised output should now look similar to Figure 2.3.

The two cells are visualised at the same time steps. Note that the dark one is deforming less and moving faster than the light one. The smaller deformation is due to its initial rotation and the faster movement is because it is located closer to the center of the channel. Think of a river, in which the water moves slowly near the banks and faster in the middle. Feel free to experiment with the simulation script, change the parameters and look at the impact your changes have on the result.

Things to ponder

What happens when the cell reaches the end of the simulation box?
What happens when you forget to specify the cell-wall interactions?
What happens when you forget to specify the cell-cell interactions?
Is it possible to move the obstacles in such a way that a cell gets trapped and does not flow forward anymore?
Can you print the cell position to the terminal as it goes? Its velocity? (The answer to this question can be found in the documentation.)

A few more comments on improving this script are in Appendix E.

2.4 Overview of the simulation module in ESPResSo

We have seen an example of what the Object-in-fluid (OIF) module can do. We will see some more in the following chapters, but here we would like to offer a more general overview. This is not a user guide with specific commands and their arguments but a brief summary of options. The actual user guide with more specifics can be found at [100].

Our aim when developing this module is that it is versatile and easy to use. The user can define cell types and then create cells, which are of these types. Both cell types and cells rely on an underlying mesh. The mesh is created using two input files, one that specifies the positions of nodes and one that specifies their incidences, i.e. which nodes form triangles together. These two files together completely characterise the geometry but not the physical properties (elasticity, viscosity) of the cell. These characteristics are entered as parameters when creating objects. While the strength of the OIF module is its capability of resolving highly elastic behavior, in principle, one can also create stiff or rigid objects.

The objects can be resized - in all, or in just some, axis directions. This is useful for scaling or for creating controlled deformities. They can also be rotated, mirrored, frozen in space or unfrozen again. Once the cells are created, we can observe their properties, such as volume, surface, extremal coordinates, largest diameter or velocity. All such information can be written as output for post-processing or visualisation.

Several analysis functions are built into our objects, too - one can examine the mesh (e.g. the average edge length, current areas of local triangular faces) or acting elastic forces (both local and global and also in the form of energy-like metric).

We can apply external force either to the whole object or just to certain mesh nodes or set the velocity of the whole object.

The objects interact with the solid boundaries of the channel using a repulsive potential and in case of periodic boundaries appear at the opposite side of the simulation box after they leave. The object position can then be tracked both folded with respect to the simulation box and unfolded.

If we use more than one cell, we can set interactions among them that use repulsive cell-cell potential based on the local outer normals to the membranes.

2.5   A few more words about simulations

While performing simulations, various reasonable practical questions start to pop up.

- **In what format should I save data?** .vtk files are all fine and good, we see them in ParaView, but most often these kinds of outputs are not what computational modelers are after. You will soon find yourself saving all kinds of other files for post-processing and/or analysis and using files like .vtk just for checks and communication of your discoveries.

- **How can I find my data once I create it?** It is good to use a sensible storage system, because just naming simulations consecutively 1, 2, 3, ..., 8345, ... is not going to cut it. A month from now, it will be impossible to tell whether simulation 123 had larger elastic coefficients than 124 and what kinds of meshes were used in simulation 42.

- **How can I reproduce my own work later if I need to?** More often than not, the word *if* in the previous sentence is a *when*. And even if that was not the case, it is always a good idea to work in such a manner that the research results are reproducible in case somebody else wants to verify them before going another step further. One way to achieve that in computational science is to save the simulation script together with the arguments passed to it.

- **What are good programming habits and tools that can help me work efficiently?** This is a great question, but unfortunately, way beyond the scope of this book. We give a few hints here and there, but we know that it is nearly not sufficient. So in parallel to reading this book it is a good idea to work on the programming skills, too.

The answers to these (and your other practical) questions are by no means easy and will require more work but what we hope to have accomplished so far is to show you that computational models are useful and that it is not too difficult to start using them.

Now with the first simulation or two under our belt, let us talk about how to develop a model of this kind. How do we match it to reality? What

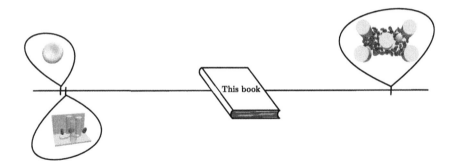

FIGURE 2.4: Right now we are on the left side of this timeline (first two bubbles) and hopefully this book can serve as a compass for navigation towards the right side.

practical issues do we need to deal with along the way? And what are the possible extensions and applications? Looking at Figure 2.4, we are at the beginning and hopefully after reading this book, we will have a consistent, working model that can also be used in applications not mentioned here. Moreover, we hope to talk about principles that will let you develop your own models and answer your own questions.

Chapter 3

Cell model

3.1   Introduction

It is very tempting to say that the most important idea to keep in mind during model development is the ability of the model to capture reality. This, however, is not completely true. We even dare to say it is *mostly* not true.

Imagine, you create a perfect model, capturing all *important* features of the modeled reality. (We have emphasised the word *important*, since we a priori assume, that the not-so-important details have been omitted and thus they do not increase the complexity of the model. Although, to recognize the distinction is also a non-trivial task.) To use the model, you need a computer implementation. This may often cause implementation problems and lead to barriers that cannot be overcome for various reasons. One can for example create a very good model, for which the accessible computational power is insufficient. Another issue is the lack of experimental data to calibrate the model.

To build a model, the following issues should be kept in mind and avoided:

- **Oversimplification:** Some of the properties of modeled objects will have to be left out for the sake of simplicity. However, it is important not to leave out any essential parts of the model, e.g. elasticity in case of red blood cells. The difficulties lie in determining what is essential and what is not. Unfortunately, by definition, here we hit a blind spot. The root cause of oversimplification is ignorance: we oversimplify when there are features or processes, which we are ignorant about. If we were not ignorant, we would include them. To know what we are ignorant about, we would need to know these facts in the first place. The Star Trek fans among us recognize the no-win Kobayashi Maru situation here. It leaves us with just one option: use the model. Use it a lot, observe and keep an open mind for the possibility that you might be wrong. Temporarily. If so, revise.

- **Overcomplication:** With the desire to build the best model out there, we might be tempted to include more and more features that will allow us to describe the system and outcome of experiments more precisely. This is like the weather forecast model that tells me the temperature for every hour of tomorrow with precision to one decimal place and the chance of rain in percent, when all I need to know when going out of the house is whether I need a jacket and/or an umbrella. Of course, an airplane pilot might need such detailed information and thus a more complicated model. Thinking about the precision of outputs should act as the stopping criterion guide for including additional complexities so that we do not end up with complexity that is not possible to embrace.

- **Unmet assumptions:** All models rely on certain assumptions. Once we try to use them in other situations or under another set of conditions, for which they were not primarily designed, it is important to review whether the assumptions still hold. Otherwise we cannot rely on the results. We must even consider assumptions that are not explicitly mentioned since they are considered too obvious.

- **Missing or impossible verification:** In physics, the criterion of veracity is experiment. If one calculates the color of gold without relativistic effects, it is silver. If the observations or results of experiments consistently contradict the theory, then the theory needs to be revised. A similar concept applies to computational models. It is essential that the models are verifiable, that experiments can be performed and that their results agree with the results obtained using the models. Also that not only can the experiments be performed, but that they actually are performed, not necessarily by us, computational scientists, but we need to actively look for them and compare to them.

This list may seem a bit daunting. On the one hand, we are not supposed to make the models too simple. On the other hand, we are not supposed to make them too complicated. While trying to strike the delicate balance between these two dangers, it is important to realise that the oversimplification is far more dangerous. The computational power keeps on increasing and from time to time catches up with the overcomplication. Even more importantly, the mistakes of omission are dangerous, not because a less precise model would just give less precise answers. They are dangerous because they might give completely wrong answers. So if unsure, try to err on the overcomplications side.

3.1.1 Biological background of the model

Let us now look at what specifically we want to model. One of the main objectives of our research is modeling blood flow considered as suspension of blood cells in blood plasma. We primarily focus on red blood cells. These cells circulate in the bloodstream and their main function is to deliver oxygen from the lungs to the peripheral tissues and to carry carbon dioxide back to the lungs. The shape of a red blood cell is a biconcave disc depicted in Figure 3.1 with a diameter of approximately $7.8\mu m$. The disc is flattened and depressed in the center, with a dumbbell-shaped cross section and with a torus-shaped rim. Its surface area for a healthy red blood cell is approximately $136\mu m^2$ and its volume is approximately $91\mu m^3$.

To serve as a carrier of the oxygen to outskirts of the circulatory system, blood cells must pass extremely thin capillaries, with cross-sections smaller than the cell diameter. Therefore, the cell membrane must be very *elastic and deformable*. Also, after such passage, the cell cannot stay deformed and has to *return to its normal shape* in order to recreate normal flow conditions in larger vessels.

The composition of red blood cells [4] is different from the majority of other cells in the body. In their mature form, they do not contain cell nuclei. These cells have nuclei during development but push them out as they mature. Mammalian red blood cells also lose all other cellular organelles such as their mitochondria, Golgi apparatus and endoplasmic reticulum. All that is left is the cell membrane and the cytoplasm.

Cytoplasm is a fairly uniform liquid rich in hemoglobin, an iron-containing biomolecule that can bind oxygen and is responsible for the red color of the cells. Oxygen and carbon dioxide can diffuse through the membrane and the red blood cells facilitate the gas exchange. The cell *keeps its volume constant* since the hemoglobin and other macromolecules are not exchanged between the cell and its surroundings.

The membrane of red blood cells with its thickness around $40 - 50nm$ is composed of a lipid bilayer with integrated proteins and an underlying spectrin network. The spectrin network is a mesh-like elastic scaffolding of interlinked proteins. To facilitate the gas exchange and functions of the plasma membrane, the density of lipids in the bilayer must be preserved and therefore the membrane must *preserve its surface area.*

Another important property of the lipid bilayer is its *viscosity* or its recip- rocal - *fluidity*. Besides lipids, the bilayer also contains some proteins and the fluidity allows these to move within the lipid bilayer.

The mesh-like structure of the spectrin network underneath the bilayer ensures that the membrane has a specific *resistance to shear deformations.*

3.1.2   Relaxed shape of the red blood cell

While there have also been a few other hypotheses proposed, the most widely used relaxed shape of the red blood cell is a biconcave discoid. A function, which describes this discoid, has been estimated, e.g. in [51], as

$$z = \pm 0.5 r_0 \left[1 - \frac{x^2 + y^2}{r_0^2} \right]^{\frac{1}{2}} \left[C_0 + C_1 \frac{x^2 + y^2}{r_0^2} + C_2 \left(\frac{x^2 + y^2}{r_0^2} \right)^2 \right], \quad (3.1)$$

where the average cell radius in the axial direction is $r_0 = 3.91 \mu m$; $[x, y, z]$ are the Cartesian coordinates and the constants are $C_0 = 0.207161$, $C_1 = 2.002558$ and $C_2 = -1.122762$.

This analytical description can be used directly in continuum models but we need to represent it by a triangular network, such as the one depicted in Figure 3.1. Triangular representation can be obtained by using various soft- wares, e.g. Gmsh [74] or Salome [165]. We discuss this in more detail in Section 5.4.3. The important point at this time is that the result of triangulation is a set of discrete points with their coordinates and a set of triangles that they form. These two sets together imply the geometrical properties of the object, such as lengths of edges or angles between triangles that enter the model in this chapter.

> **What is triangulation?**
> Triangulation of a surface means a net of triangles, which approximately covers the surface. The vertices of the triangles are located on the trian- gulated surface.

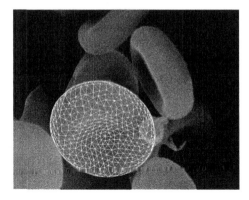

FIGURE 3.1: Micrograph of red blood cells with a triangular mesh overlay. Adapted from [8].

3.1.3 Mechanics defined by biology

In Section 3.1.1, we have *emphasised* several properties of the cell. Although these properties were derived from the biological functions and composition of the cell structures, they are all of a mechanical nature. Let us summarise:

- Membrane is elastic and deformable

- Membrane tends to return to its original shape even after severe deformation

- Membrane encapsulates fluid with fixed volume

- Membrane has a constant surface area

- Membrane has a resistance to shear deformations

These biological properties have their mechanical counterparts in the theory of thin sheet materials. Mechanically, the bilayer is responsible for the membrane surface incompressibility, provides bending resistance and is viscous while the spectrin layer provides resistance mainly to the in-plane membrane shearing [116]. More detailed explanation of these terms is given in Section 4.2.1.

Due to their physical similarity, spring network models have been used to imitate the function of the spectrin network underlying the red cell membrane. The stretching of individual edges in the spring network - they are effectively functioning as springs - resembles the in-plane membrane shearing. This defines one of the moduli and is called *stretching modulus.*

The mechanical properties of the lipid bilayer can be modeled by spring networks as well. The bilayer allows the membrane to bend and to relax and this can be controlled by enforcing the preferred angles between the neighboring triangles in the mesh. This mechanism functions as springs between pairs of adjacent triangles and is called *bending modulus*. The bilayer also mediates the membrane surface incompressibility. This is modeled by *local area modulus*. The last phenomenon that is caused by the structure of the bilayer is membrane viscosity. This contribution is called *viscosity modulus*.

The viscosity modulus is slightly different than the other moduli mentioned so far because instead of conserving any geometrical characteristics, it conserves *state*. It makes the object resist change - the faster the change, the more resistance the modulus puts up.

So far, we have described the microscopic mechanical properties of the spectrin network and lipid bilayer. There are also macroscopic properties that are linked to the fact that the cell is a three-dimensional object enclosed by its membrane. Thus the volume and the surface of the cell remain fairly constant. This phenomenon has to be captured by macroscopic mechanisms, since the local elements of the membrane do not have any information about the global volume or global surface. The elastic modulus responsible for preserving global surface is called *global area modulus* and the one responsible for volume conservation is called *volume modulus*.

All of these moduli work toward reducing the effect of any deformation by bringing the cell back to its resting shape. As shown in [80], red blood cells assume several mechanically stable shapes, which can also be derived using membrane mechanics and material-parameter inputs, however, the basic steady resting shape of a mature healthy red blood cell (RBC) is a biconcave discoid, as depicted in Figure 3.1.

What are spring network and elastic moduli?

A *spring network*, or *spring system*, is a model of physics composed of several points defined by their physical positions in three-dimensional space and by springs between some pairs of the points. The springs have a given stiffness and according to the current physical position of the points, each spring exerts forces on the end points of the spring. We work mostly with spring networks resembling two-dimensional (2D) surfaces enclosing three-dimensional (3D) objects. In these cases, the spring network points are distributed on the surface of a 3D object and the springs link the points that are next to each other on the surface.

The well-known notion of a *spring between two points* may be generalised. For example, instead of a metal spring with two ends, imagine a circular rubber band wrapped around three points. If you pull these three points apart, the rubber band extends and exerts a force on all three points simultaneously. This force depends on the total prolongation of the rubber band and thus the force is defined by the relative position of the three points. This is an example of a *spring among three points.* In a similar manner, one can extend this notion to a *spring among four points.* We do not consider generalisations beyond that.

A spring network with one set of points may have different types of springs. For example, we can have several pairs of points connected by thin metal springs, several pairs connected by thick metal springs and several rubber bands wrapped around triplets of points. Some points may be connected to one or more thin or thick metal springs and to one or even more rubber bands.

Each such type of springs may have a common formula for computation of the force exerted on the end points (two, three or four). The formula typically consists of mathematical expressions involving position vectors of the corresponding points. Besides that, the formula contains a pre-factor, a linear scaling, that determines the strength of the forces or, when speaking about the springs, their stiffness. This pre-factor is called *elastic modulus.*

We also use the term *elastic modulus* when we refer to the types of the springs. In the example above, we would have three different elastic moduli - thin metal springs, thick metal springs and rubber bands - each type with its own formula and pre-factor.

3.1.4 Components of the fluid-cell model

The focus of our research is modeling of cell flow on the level of individual cells. Our approach was to have the fluid and cells computed by two principally different methods, which are coupled to ensure a proper interaction between cells and fluid. We thus have three main building blocks: fluid solver, cell model and fluid-cell coupling.

This approach has several advantages:

- It has allowed us to leave the development of the fluidic part to other experts, choose from the available fluid solvers and focus on the cell.

- In case we decide later to use a different method for fluidic computations instead of the currently used lattice-Boltzmann method, we can do so quite easily without significant changes to the cell model.

- Moreover, we can even alter the current method for the cell-fluid coupling and instead of dissipative coupling explained later in Section 3.5, we can use, e.g. immersed boundary method or another boundary tracking method.

A short introduction and a few details on the lattice-Boltzmann method are in Section 3.5.1. The scope of this book is however on cell modeling and we leave the detailed description of the fluidic part to specialised works such as [109]. The coupling of both methods is thoroughly analysed in Section 3.5.

For modeling of the cell we have used the spring network model. It is based on a triangular mesh covering the surface of the cell. The surface is discretised using mesh points and the mechano-elastic properties of the membrane are represented by different types of bonds and forces between neighboring mesh points. This way, the deformation of the object changes the relaxed distances between the mesh points and this induces forces acting against these changes. The forces cause the mesh points to move in space and thus the temporal changes of the cell's shape are computed from Newton's equations of motion given the deformation forces for each mesh point. This approach allows further extensions by adding inner parts of the cell, such as nucleus, into the model.

Force-based approach
In the physical world, mechanical actions and reactions are mediated by forces. Our cell model is based on mechanics and we use forces for all phenomena that we take into consideration.

   This is not the only possible approach (and we briefly mention other options) but it is quite flexible. Should the membrane stretch? Then we apply forces to the membrane discretisation points causing this stretching. Should the membrane flow around an obstacle? Then we apply forces (to the membrane discretisation points) preventing the membrane from intersecting with obstacle boundaries. Should the fluid deform the membrane? Then we apply forces (again to the membrane discretisation points) in the direction of the fluid effectively deforming the membrane.

Mesh and related concepts
Membrane - A biological cell membrane is an elastic 2D surface enclosing inner parts of a cell. It is composed of a lipid bilayer with proteins supported by a spectrin scaffolding-like structure on the inside.
Spring network again - Model representation of the membrane, consisting of connected springs that form a network. The network may or may not be regular. While it resembles the spectrin network of the biological membrane, it is coarser and it is meant to capture the mechanical properties of both the spectrin network and the lipid bilayer.
Elastic and viscous forces - Forces acting in the spectrin network to model the deformability of the membrane.
Mesh - Computational representation of the spring network, typically triangular, given by a set of (mesh) points, often called vertices, and triangles they form.
Mesh point - A basic component of mesh. Two neighboring mesh points are connected by an edge. Each edge is adjacent to exactly two triangles. The triangles form a closed surface - mesh. In practice, these mesh points are particles that have mass and they move according to Newton's equations of motion as driven by forces. Note that in some literature, the term *particle* is also used to denote a cell or a capsule - a whole object in flow.

> *Relaxed state* - The initial relative placement of mesh components (mesh points, angles, edges, triangles) defining its relaxed state. Any deformation from this state causes forces that act to restore it.

3.1.5 Classification of elastic forces

Models in general are often created by putting together several concepts - in our case various forces - that all seem to be crucial but sometimes appear unrelated at first glance. Therefore, we start here with a classification of forces to help us understand their properties better and to look at their similarities and differences.

The first classification is fairly straightforward. It concerns the range of interactions represented by the forces. We can divide these interactions into two categories: local and global. In our case, the local interactions include the stretching, bending, local area and viscosity moduli. All of these forces describe phenomena with spatially limited ranges and can be defined locally. Global interactions represent the processes that involve the cell as a whole: global area and volume conservation moduli.

For a simpler analysis of a continuous mechanics model of thin membranes, the majority of authors decompose the membrane elastic forces into their normal components and tangential components. These components are also called *out-of-plane* and *in-plane* contributions. Since the spring network is a spatial discretisation, we do not know the tangents and the normals at the vertices. Therefore, we use normals and tangents to the triangles. In the spring network analysis we follow this decomposition and we distinguish between the forces that are applied in the plane of the mesh triangles and the forces that point in the normal directions to those triangles.

These two classifications are motivated by biomechanics. There are, however, some other basic rules for spring network models that apply generally, regardless of the application field.

> **Momentum conservation**
> If an object modeled by a spring network is not under an influence of any external forces, it should neither move nor rotate in the absence of initial velocity and torque.

The momentum conservation requirements are completely natural and should be fulfilled by any spring network model. The requirements themselves are often called *force-free* and *torque-free* conditions. Following these terms, one can introduce two more classifications: one distinguishing between elastic moduli that are or are not force-free, and one that recognizes, whether they are or are not torque-free.

	stretching	bending	local area	global area	volume	viscosity
local/global	local	local	local	global	global	local
in/out of plane	in	?	in	?	?	?
force-free?	yes	?	?	?	?	?
torque-free?	yes	?	?	?	?	?

TABLE 3.1: Categorisations of elastic moduli - first guess

To summarise, we now have four different categorisations of our moduli:

- Local vs. global

- In-plane vs. out-of-plane

- Force-free vs. non-force-free

- Torque-free vs. non-torque-free

From the information about the six elastic moduli provided so far, one can guess some characteristics. In Table 3.1, we can see that it is easy to categorise the moduli by the first property. For the remaining three, the classification depends on the actual implementation of the underlying forces. The stretching modulus is the simplest and we can decide all categories: It is a local, in-plane, force- and torque-free contribution to elasticity. For local area, we can safely say that it is in-plane, since the triangle shrinking or expansion is certainly done in the plane of the triangle. However, the other relations cannot be decided at this stage.

In this chapter, we fill in the remaining fields in this table and discuss the outcomes. Ideally, we would like to have all *yes-es* in the last two rows.

Note that in this approach, we directly prescribe the forces responsible for the six elastic moduli: stretching, bending, local area, global area, volume preservation and viscosity modulus. Some other possibilities, such as models derived from membrane energetics, will be mentioned later.

Properties of elastic moduli

in-plane - The vector of an in-plane elastic force is in the plane of the surface triangle, to which it belongs.

out-of-plane - The vector of an out-of-plane elastic force is not in the plane of the surface triangle, to which it belongs. Typically, we consider such a vector to be perpendicular to the triangle plane, since otherwise it could be decomposed into its in-plane and perpendicular components.

force-free - Due to momentum conservation, the resultant of all forces generated by elastic modulus must be zero.

torque-free - Similarly, the resultant of all torques must be zero.

3.2 Local membrane mechanics

The microstructure of the membrane defines how the membrane behaves locally and this behavior can be captured by defining the interactions between neighboring elements of the mesh (e.g. two points of an edge, three points forming a triangle and four points forming two adjacent triangles).

Stretching modulus

When a piece of cell membrane is stretched it develops resistance against this stretching. To translate such resistance into elastic stretching of individual mesh edges in a spring network, we implement a spring with relaxed length and non-linear stiffness law by

$$\mathbf{F}_s(A) = k_s \kappa(\lambda)(L - L_0)\mathbf{p}_{AB} \tag{3.2}$$

where k_s is a stretching coefficient, L_0 and L are the relaxed length and the current length of the edge AB, $\mathbf{p}_{AB}$ is a unit vector pointing from A to B and non-linear function $\kappa(\lambda)$ models neo-Hookean non-linearity of the stretching force by

$$\lambda = \frac{L}{L_0} \quad \text{and} \quad \kappa(\lambda) = \frac{\lambda^{0.5} + \lambda^{-2.5}}{\lambda + \lambda^{-3}}.$$

Expression (3.2) generates force applied at mesh point A that shrinks the edge AB when $L > L_0$ and extends it when $L < L_0$, Figure 3.2. An opposite force is applied at vertex B.

Neo-Hookean model

Hooke's law is the principle of physics, which states that the force needed to extend (or contract) a spring is proportional to the extension (contraction), i.e. that we have a linear relationship.

The neo-Hookean model is an extension of this law to situations that involve substances like rubber or polymers. If those are stretched, we initially observe a linear relationship, however at a certain point we encounter a non-linearity. This is due to the fact that polymer chains can initially move relative to one another fairly easily, but once the extension reaches their bond lengths, there is a significant increase in the elastic modulus of the material. Similarly, the molecules can only be comfortably packed to some extent, further compression requires much larger stress. Cell membranes are composed of macromolecules and thus a neo-Hookean model is much more suitable than a linear one. The specific form of the non-linearity has been taken from [48].

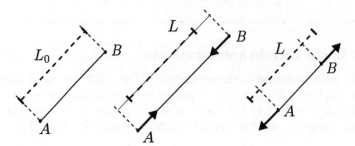

FIGURE 3.2: Stretching force. If $L > L_0$, opposite non-linear forces act to contract the edge AB. If $L < L_0$, they act to expand it. At rest, $L = L_0$ and no stretching forces are applied.

Stretching is force- and torque-free

Although κ in (3.2) makes this elastic modulus non-linear, it is the same for $\mathbf{F}_s(A)$ and $\mathbf{F}_s(B)$. Therefore, even non-linear stretching contribution is force-free: $\mathbf{F}_s(A) + \mathbf{F}_s(B) = \mathbf{F}_s(A) - \mathbf{F}_s(A) = \mathbf{0}$.

Also, the torque-free condition holds directly

$$\mathbf{r}_A \times \mathbf{F}_s(A) + \mathbf{r}_B \times \mathbf{F}_s(B) = \mathbf{r}_A \times \mathbf{F}_s(A) + (\mathbf{r}_A + (\mathbf{B} - \mathbf{A})) \times \mathbf{F}_s(B)$$
$$= \mathbf{r}_A \times \mathbf{F}_s(A) - \mathbf{r}_A \times \mathbf{F}_s(A) + (\mathbf{B} - \mathbf{A}) \times \mathbf{F}_s(B)$$
$$= (\mathbf{B} - \mathbf{A}) \times \mathbf{F}_s(B) = \mathbf{0}.$$

The last equality holds because the vectors $(\mathbf{B} - \mathbf{A})$ and $\mathbf{F}_s(B)$ are colinear. Vectors $\mathbf{r}_A$, $\mathbf{r}_B$ point from an arbitrary point in space to points A and B, respectively.

Bending modulus

The biological membrane of a red blood cell is flexible and can bend quite easily. The resistance is relatively weak, but the membrane still generates forces acting against the bending. Consider a membrane bent in such a way that locally it resembles a part of a sphere. In such a case, the smaller the radius of the sphere, the greater are the forces resisting the bending. The inverse value of the radius of the inscribed sphere represents a *local curvature* of the membrane and tells us about the resistance we encounter in bending.

To introduce bending resistance into the spring network, we use angles between neighboring triangles in a mesh. In equilibrium, the spring network has a prescribed *relaxed state* with relaxed angles between neighboring triangles. Bending forces act towards preserving the relaxed angle. Given coordinates of four vertices forming two triangles with a common edge, one can compute the angle between the triangles. However, without any further information, it is not possible to distinguish between the angle or its complement to 2π.

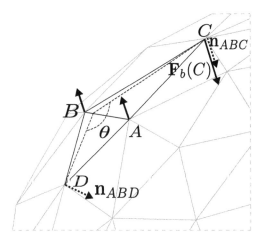

FIGURE 3.3: Orientations of two adjacent triangles in a mesh with normal vectors as dotted arrows.

We need to introduce the orientation of the triangles. Assume two adjacent triangles, ABC and ABD, with common edge AB and other two vertices C and D. Here we need to know, which way is inside and which way outside of the cell, when these triangles are on its surface. Therefore, we compute the normal vectors to triangles ABC and ABD by

$$\mathbf{n}_{ABC} = \frac{(\mathbf{B} - \mathbf{C}) \times (\mathbf{A} - \mathbf{C})}{|(\mathbf{B} - \mathbf{C}) \times (\mathbf{A} - \mathbf{C})|}, \quad \mathbf{n}_{ABD} = \frac{(\mathbf{A} - \mathbf{D}) \times (\mathbf{B} - \mathbf{D})}{|(\mathbf{A} - \mathbf{D}) \times (\mathbf{B} - \mathbf{D})|},$$

and we assume that both normal vectors point towards the inside of the cell, see Figure 3.3. The bending force applied at vertex C is then given by

$$\mathbf{F}_b(C) = k_b(\theta - \theta_0)\mathbf{n}_{ABC}, \tag{3.3}$$

(Warning: This formula will eventually
be changed later!)

where k_b is the bending coefficient, θ_0 and θ are the resting angle and the current angle between two triangles that have common edge AB. An analogous force with the corresponding normal vector $\mathbf{n}_{ABD}$ is applied at vertex D. To keep the contribution of bending forces force-free, we apply one half of $\mathbf{F}_b(C)$ and $\mathbf{F}_b(D)$ with minus sign to both vertices A and B, see Figure 3.4.

Characteristics of bending forces
Given the formula for the bending force, we can try to fill in some information into Table 3.1. From the way we have defined $\mathbf{F}_b(A)$ and $\mathbf{F}_b(B)$, it is clear that the resultant of bending forces corresponding to triangles

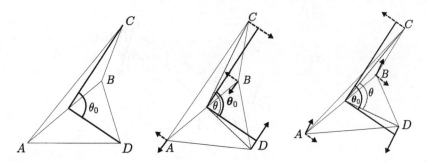

FIGURE 3.4: Bending forces act to restore the relaxed angle θ_0 between two adjacent triangles.

ABC and ABD is zero. To analyse the effect of bending modulus on an object, it is important to realise that the object is enclosed by a surface covered by a triangular mesh. Such a mesh has the property that each edge belongs to two triangles and thus the bending contribution at each vertex is calculated as a sum of bending forces corresponding to all its edges. Therefore, the resultant force on the whole object is also zero and the bending modulus is force-free with respect to the whole object, as well as with respect to any edge.

The bending forces are always applied along the normals to the triangles, so the bending modulus is an out-of-plane contribution.

The question whether the bending modulus is torque-free is not so easy to answer, but the computation of the torque reveals that the bending forces defined in (3.3) do not meet the torque-free condition. For now, we omit these computations but we return to this topic in Section 3.4.

Local area modulus

The lipid bilayer consists of densely packed lipids. The lipids *stick* together and thus they do not allow the bilayer to change its surface area much.

To mimic this behavior, we use a mechanism to preserve the area of triangles forming the triangular spring network. This mechanism generates forces for each triangle, which we call *local area forces*.

Denote by T the centroid of the triangle ABC and by $\mathbf{t}_A, \mathbf{t}_B, \mathbf{t}_C$ denote the vectors AT, BT and CT. Then the definition of local area force applied to vertex A is given by

$$\mathbf{F}_{al}(A) = k_{al} \frac{S - S_0}{|\mathbf{t}_A|^2 + |\mathbf{t}_B|^2 + |\mathbf{t}_C|^2} \mathbf{t}_A, \qquad (3.4)$$

where k_{al} is the local area coefficient, S_0 and S are the relaxed area and

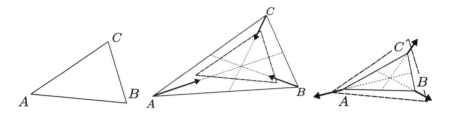

FIGURE 3.5: Proportional local area force.

current area of triangle ABC. Analogous forces are assigned to vertices B and C.

This implementation functions well: If the current triangle area is larger than the relaxed area, the triangle tries to shrink and vice versa as depicted in Figure 3.5. However, the formula is purely phenomenological. It does not follow from any biological reasoning, unlike the definition of stretching forces, where the springs *mimic* the spectrin filaments. Therefore, we have multiple choices how to implement such behavior. We could have picked different directions of the forces: Instead of medians we could have taken altitudes of the triangle. Such an approach was used in [56]. Or, we could have left the force directions along the medians but picked different weighting factors. In [48], the distribution of the local area forces is equal among the three triangle vertices.

We have discussed this issue in more detail in [102], where we have concluded that first, equal force distribution results in non-force-free implementation of local area forces. Second, we have shown that while the approach in [56] is force-free, when a triangle becomes obtuse then even if the relaxed triangle is acute, such a definition of local area forces prefers further growth of the obtuse angle. And finally, we have proven that our formula (3.4) gives force-free and torque-free contributions.

Characteristics of local area forces

We can now fill in some more fields in Table 3.1. The local area forces are applied in the triangle's plane so this contribution is in-plane. As we have discussed, they are force-free and torque-free.

The local area formula (3.4) was not like this at the beginning. Our first attempt was to use the formula:

$$k_{al} \frac{S - S_0}{S_0} \frac{\mathbf{t}_A}{|\mathbf{t}_A|}.$$

Here, the direction of the force is the same, from the vertex towards the centroid. The amplitude of the force is the same for all vertices of the triangle and depends on the relative deviation of the triangle's surface. This practically means that the units for coefficient k_{al} are newtons and this does not correspond to any physically relevant mechanical quantities, such as Young's modulus or area compressibility modulus. We have quickly realised this and rectified this inconsistency in the model by using normalisation by length instead of by area:

$$k_{al}\frac{S - S_0}{\sqrt{S_0}}\frac{\mathbf{t}_A}{|\mathbf{t}_A|}.$$

Only after some time, we have changed the formula again, in order to shrink or enlarge the triangle isometrically. We have divided the local area force among the three vertices according to the lengths of the corresponding medians (3.4). This has also had the effect that the formula became force-free and torque-free, which was not the case for the previous two attempts.

Viscosity modulus

Lipids present in the membrane can move within the bilayer. The membrane is thus fluidic and similarly to liquids, has a resistance against shearing. This resistance is called *viscosity*.

To consider the viscosity of the membrane, we employ the Kelvin-Voigt model. For a simple oscillator, this model consists of a Newtonian damper connected to a spring in parallel [130]. In our case of spring network, the damper must act against the relative movement of the mesh points and must be proportional to their relative velocities. For viscosity modulus, the viscous forces are defined as

$$\mathbf{F}_{visc}(A) = -k_{visc}\frac{dL}{dt} = -k_{visc}(\mathbf{v}_{AB}, \mathbf{p}_{AB})\mathbf{p}_{AB}, \qquad (3.5)$$

where k_{visc} is the viscosity coefficient, L is the distance between A and B, d/dt denotes time derivative, $\mathbf{v}_{AB}$ denotes relative velocity of mesh points A and B and $\mathbf{p}_{AB}$ is the unit directional vector between A, B, see Figure 3.6. Analogous force with the opposite sign is assigned to vertex B.

Characteristics of viscous forces
Since the viscous forces are assigned along the mesh edges, the contribution is in-plane. Analogically to the stretching modulus, opposite forces along an edge cancel out and thus the contribution is force-free and torque-free.

To understand the formula (3.5) better, we can look at Figure 3.7. The viscosity modulus does not use the velocity difference vector $\mathbf{v}$ directly, but its projection on the vector $\mathbf{p}$, which connects the two points A, B. To find the projection $\mathbf{a}$, consider the angle φ between the vectors $\mathbf{v}$ and $\mathbf{p}$. On the

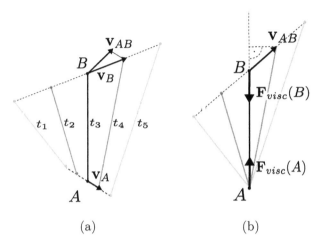

(a)   (b)

FIGURE 3.6: Viscous forces. Magnitude of viscous forces is proportional to the relative velocity $\mathbf{v}_{AB}$ of two points connected by an edge. The direction of viscous force is along the edge and acts against the projection of the velocity difference vector. (a) Movement of edge AB in five different time instances $t_1, \ldots, t_5$ represented by the greyscale tones. (b) Relative movement of B with respect to A.

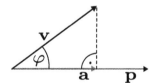

FIGURE 3.7: Projection $\mathbf{a}$ of a vector $\mathbf{v}$ onto another vector: $\mathbf{p}$.

one hand, this angle can be computed from the dot product as

$$\cos(\varphi) = \frac{(\mathbf{v}, \mathbf{p})}{|\mathbf{v}||\mathbf{p}|}.$$

On the other hand, the same angle can be expressed using trigonometry in the right triangle as

$$\cos(\varphi) = \frac{|\mathbf{a}|}{|\mathbf{v}|}.$$

By equating these two expressions we get

$$|\mathbf{a}| = \frac{(\mathbf{v}, \mathbf{p})}{|\mathbf{p}|}.$$

We know that the direction of $\mathbf{a}$ is the same as the direction of $\mathbf{p}$ and moreover, in our case $\mathbf{p}$ is a unit vector. Therefore, we can write:

$$\mathbf{a} = (\mathbf{v}, \mathbf{p})\mathbf{p},$$

which is the vector in formula (3.5).

3.3　Global membrane mechanics

Unlike the local interactions, global interactions capture phenomena that are not linked directly to the microstructure of the membrane. The physically relevant property of the cell is that the cell keeps its volume and surface fairly constant under constant osmotic conditions. This property has to be implemented phenomenologically and most approaches use a simple idea:

> **Phenomenological approach to global forces**
> If the cell's surface is larger than desired, try to decrease it. If it is smaller, try to increase it. The same idea is used for the volume.

Global area modulus

Motivated by the formula for local area forces, we have suggested the global area forces as

$$\mathbf{F}_{ag}(A) = k_{ag} \frac{S^c - S_0^c}{|\mathbf{t}_A|^2 + |\mathbf{t}_B|^2 + |\mathbf{t}_C|^2} \mathbf{t}_A, \tag{3.6}$$

(Warning: This formula will eventually
be changed later!)

where k_{ag} is the global area coefficient and superscript ^{c} stands for *cell*. S^c and S_0^c denote the current and relaxed surface of the whole cell.

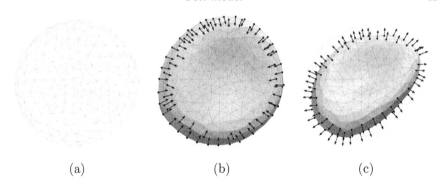

(a)   (b)   (c)

FIGURE 3.8: Volume forces depicted on the outer rim of the cell: (a) Relaxed shape represented by wireframe, no forces present. (b) Cell is expanded from the relaxed shape, forces point inwards. (c) Cell is deformed in such a way that volume is slightly lower than in relaxed shape, forces point outwards.

Characteristics of global area forces
This implementation is force-free and torque-free and since the forces are applied in the triangle's plane, it belongs to the in-plane contributions.

Things to ponder
A natural question to ask is, why do we need both local and global area conservation?
Why is it not enough to have the local elastic moduli, which already include local area forces, and complement them with volume conservation?
What happens in the simulation, when we set k_{ag} (only k_{ag}) to 0?

The answer to the previous questions is that perhaps in simulations of natural processes this might not be such an issue, but in simulations of cell manipulations, such as the stretching experiment using optical tweezers discussed and illustrated in Section 4.3.1, when locally the triangles deform significantly, we still need the cell to maintain its global surface (and volume).

Volume modulus

This modulus phenomenologically deals with an object's resistance to uniform compression or expansion. The formula for volume forces is

$$\mathbf{F}_V = -k_v \frac{V^c - V_0^c}{V_0^c} S_{ABC} \mathbf{n}_{ABC}, \tag{3.7}$$

where k_v is the volume coefficient, V^c and V_0^c are volumes of the cell in the current and in the relaxed shape, and $\mathbf{n}_{ABC}$ is the unit normal vector to the

	stretching	bending	local area	global area	volume	viscosity
local/global	local	local	local	global	global	local
in/out of plane	in	out	in	in	out	in
force-free?	yes	yes	yes	yes	yes	yes
torque-free?	yes	no	yes	yes	yes	yes

TABLE 3.2: Categorisations of elastic moduli - completed

plane ABC. This force corresponds to one triangle and therefore it is divided by three and then applied to vertices of the triangle. Direction of the force is along the triangle's normal vector pointing inside the cell, see Figure 3.8.

Characteristics of volume forces

The volume forces are perpendicular to the triangles, so we classify them as out-of-plane contribution. Force-free and torque-free conditions for volume forces can be verified by computations presented in Appendix C.1.

Things to ponder

Why do the elastic coefficients have different units?

Note that the stretching and local/global area coefficients have units $[N/m]$, while the global volume coefficient has units $[N/m^2]$. This is due to the fact that in-plane elasticity essentially works as force per length. We can think of it as stretching a piece of cloth or balloon membrane in our hands. The volume force has to be considered per (unit of) area, which means m^2 in the denominator. This idea also translates into bending elasticity. Here the force needs to be per unit of angle, which is dimensionless and thus the coefficient has units just $[N]$.

Another thing worth noticing is that the multiplication by the area S_{ABC} in the equation (3.7) in a way corresponds to the multiplication by length $|\mathbf{t}_A|$ in the equation (3.4). This proportionality in the distribution of forces ensures that the shape restoring elastic forces maintain congruent shape of the object and do not cause extreme local changes. This topic will be discussed in more detail in Section 3.4.

Now that we have discussed all elastic (and viscous) interactions, we can fill in Table 3.1 and we get Table 3.2. It looks almost perfect. The only flaw is the torque-free condition, which is not satisfied for the bending modulus. This is kind of suspicious. We were able to adapt the local area modulus from the expression $k_{al}\frac{S-S_0}{\sqrt{S_0}}$ that was not torque-free to (3.4), which is. The global area modulus followed the path of the local area modulus. The volume was the most challenging because of its non-local character, but apparently it can also be done in a torque-free fashion. So what is the problem with the bending modulus? Is it really not possible to make it torque-free?

A look at other approaches (more details can be found in Section 3.7.2) shows that it indeed should be possible. A new visit of the bending interaction is in order.

3.4 Membrane mechanics revisited

While the previous section shows a reasonable model and the rationale behind its development, here we would like to address a few more delicate issues that we have skipped over. The first and the most important one is the desire to make the bending modulus torque-free. After that, we return to the proportionality in the distribution of forces and issues with in-plane and out-of-plane forces.

3.4.1 How to make bending torque-free?

First things first, how do we know that the bending modulus as defined by (3.3) is not torque-free? We calculate the torque of the four-point interaction using the notation from Figure 3.3 and denoting R the centroid of the four-point object. For $\mathbf{T}_{ABC}, \mathbf{T}_{ABD}$, the respective torques of triangles ABC and ABD, we get

$$
\begin{aligned}
\mathbf{T}_{ABC} &= (\mathbf{A} - \mathbf{R}) \times (-\tfrac{1}{2}\mathbf{F}_C) + (\mathbf{B} - \mathbf{R}) \times (-\tfrac{1}{2}\mathbf{F}_C) + (\mathbf{C} - \mathbf{R}) \times \mathbf{F}_C \\
&= (-\tfrac{1}{2}\mathbf{A} - \tfrac{1}{2}\mathbf{B} + \mathbf{C}) \times \mathbf{F}_C.
\end{aligned}
$$

Similarly we have

$$
\begin{aligned}
\mathbf{T}_{ABD} &= (\mathbf{A} - \mathbf{R}) \times (-\tfrac{1}{2}\mathbf{F}_D) + (\mathbf{B} - \mathbf{R}) \times (-\tfrac{1}{2}\mathbf{F}_D) + (\mathbf{D} - \mathbf{R}) \times \mathbf{F}_D \\
&= (-\tfrac{1}{2}\mathbf{A} - \tfrac{1}{2}\mathbf{B} + \mathbf{D}) \times \mathbf{F}_D.
\end{aligned}
$$

While in some special situations these two contributions might cancel out, in general they do not. We have approached this issue pragmatically: Let us change the (reasonably well-working) formulas in some way so that they become torque-free. We keep the features that work, and we modify those that do not. Which features work?

- *Being out-of-plane*

- *Being force-free*

The first requirement is easy to meet. We keep the bending forces perpendicular to triangles they are assigned to. Since the basic task for the bending forces is to act by increasing or decreasing the angle between two adjacent triangles when disturbed from their relaxed position, we also keep the directions of the bending forces as depicted in Figure 3.3.

To conform to the second requirement, we need to make sure that the sum of the forces in one triangle vanishes. For example, in triangle ABC, the forces in A and B have the opposite direction as the force in C. The condition $\mathbf{F}_A + \mathbf{F}_B + \mathbf{F}_C = 0$ leaves us with only one free parameter k (in the original definition we had $k = 1/2$):

$$\mathbf{F}_A = -k\mathbf{F}_C, \quad \mathbf{F}_B = -(1-k)\mathbf{F}_C.$$

Similarly, in triangle ABD, we get another free parameter l by defining

$$\mathbf{F}_A = -l\mathbf{F}_D, \quad \mathbf{F}_B = -(1-l)\mathbf{F}_D.$$

Using the two free parameters k and l we have some freedom in defining the bending forces while preserving the force-free condition and out-of-plane property. We can express the torque exerted on the two triangles and try to set k and l in such a way that the torque vanishes. It turns out, it is possible by choosing

$$k = \frac{(\mathbf{A} - \mathbf{B}, \mathbf{C} - \mathbf{B})}{(\mathbf{A} - \mathbf{B}, \mathbf{A} - \mathbf{B})} \quad \text{and} \quad l = \frac{(\mathbf{A} - \mathbf{B}, \mathbf{D} - \mathbf{B})}{(\mathbf{A} - \mathbf{B}, \mathbf{A} - \mathbf{B})}$$

and the magnitudes of forces $\mathbf{F}_C$ and $\mathbf{F}_D$ that fulfil

$$\frac{|\mathbf{F}_C|}{|\mathbf{F}_D|} = \frac{S_{ABD}}{S_{ABC}}.$$

Detailed derivation of force expressions is presented in Appendix A.1 and A.3. Here we sum up relations involving position vectors $\mathbf{A}, \mathbf{B}, \mathbf{C}$ and $\mathbf{D}$:

$$
\begin{aligned}
\mathbf{F}_A &= -k_b(\theta - \theta_0)\left(\frac{\mathbf{N}_C}{|\mathbf{N}_C|^2} \frac{(\mathbf{A} - \mathbf{B}, \mathbf{C} - \mathbf{B})}{|\mathbf{B} - \mathbf{A}|} + \frac{\mathbf{N}_D}{|\mathbf{N}_D|^2} \frac{(\mathbf{A} - \mathbf{B}, \mathbf{D} - \mathbf{B})}{|\mathbf{B} - \mathbf{A}|} \right) \\
\mathbf{F}_B &= -k_b(\theta - \theta_0)\left(\frac{\mathbf{N}_C}{|\mathbf{N}_C|^2} \frac{(\mathbf{A} - \mathbf{B}, \mathbf{A} - \mathbf{D})}{|\mathbf{B} - \mathbf{A}|} + \frac{\mathbf{N}_D}{|\mathbf{N}_D|^2} \frac{(\mathbf{A} - \mathbf{B}, \mathbf{D} - \mathbf{B})}{|\mathbf{B} - \mathbf{A}|} \right) \\
\mathbf{F}_C &= k_b(\theta - \theta_0)|\mathbf{B} - \mathbf{A}|\frac{\mathbf{N}_C}{|\mathbf{N}_C|^2} \\
\mathbf{F}_D &= k_b(\theta - \theta_0)|\mathbf{B} - \mathbf{A}|\frac{\mathbf{N}_D}{|\mathbf{N}_D|^2}
\end{aligned}
\tag{3.8}
$$

where $\mathbf{N}_C = (\mathbf{A} - \mathbf{C}) \times (\mathbf{B} - \mathbf{C})$ is normal vector to ABC and $\mathbf{N}_D = (\mathbf{B} - \mathbf{D}) \times (\mathbf{A} - \mathbf{D})$ is normal vetor to ABD.

We further show in Appendix A.2 how the effort to make the bending modulus torque-free has resulted in a unification of our approach with other similar approaches for modeling of bending. For a more detailed discussion of modeling of bending, we refer the reader to the work [82].

Without any further complaints, we can finalize Table 3.3.

	stretching	bending	local area	global area	volume	viscosity
local/global	local	local	local	global	global	local
in/out of plane	in	out	in	in	out	in
force-free?	yes	yes	yes	yes	yes	yes
torque-free?	yes	yes	yes	yes	yes	yes

TABLE 3.3: Categorisations of elastic moduli - final.

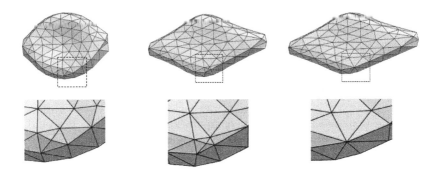

FIGURE 3.9: Annihilation of triangles due to comparatively large local contributions of global area force.

3.4.2 Triangle annihilation and its implications for global area force

Let us now consider the differences between the two global forces - conservation of volume and conservation of global area, equations (3.6) and (3.7). The global area force calculates the absolute difference of current and relaxed surface of the object and then proportionally divides the elastic force among the triangle nodes. The volume force calculates the relative difference of the current and global volume and weights it by the triangle area.

In the former case, a situation may arise, in which some triangles have significantly different area than others, if part of the object is significantly deformed, while the rest of it is undisturbed. This may result in small triangles receiving disproportionately large force contributions that cause them to shrink even further. In extreme cases, we may also see a triangle annihilation as depicted in Figure 3.9.

To avoid this, we have included a scaling term, area of the triangle, into the definition of global area force, see (3.9). With this factor, we no longer have triangle annihilation and the force- and torque-free conditions still hold:

$$\mathbf{F}_{ag}(A) = k_{ag} \frac{S^c - S_0^c}{S_0^c} S_{ABC} \frac{\mathbf{t}_A}{|\mathbf{t}_A|^2 + |\mathbf{t}_B|^2 + |\mathbf{t}_C|^2}. \tag{3.9}$$

3.4.3 Competing in-plane and not-out-of-plane moduli and implications for volume force

Suppose we use a volume force analogous to area forces - acting towards the centroid of the object and thus not locally perpendicular to surface triangles. This is a natural extension of the same principle we have used in the area forces. It would have the same advantage of proportional distribution of forces: The points that are further away from the centroid, would get a larger volume force contribution compared to the points that are closer. Consequently, the the shrinking/expansion (in the absence of other forces) would result in congruent objects. This approach is technically possible and seemingly logically sound, however, it has two major drawbacks.

The first one is increase in computational complexity. It would require three loops over the cell particles (one to calculate centroid and current volume, second to calculate node distances to centroid to be used as weights and third to calculate the proportional forces) compared to two loops needed for the volume force defined by (3.7) (one to calculate the current volume and second to calculate the volume forces). This might not seem too bad until we consider that these calculations are done for each cell at each time step.

The second reason is that in this case, the volume forces would not be locally perpendicular to the planes of individual triangles. Instead, they would point either to or from the centroid of the whole object. As a consequence, they would in general have a non-zero in-plane component, that would be effectively added to the global area forces. This could be problematic if the two were in competition.

Consider a model situation like the one depicted in Figure 3.10 (a). We have an elastic sphere with radius $r = 1$ that is deformed into an ellipsoid with semiaxes $a = 1.9$ and $b = c = 0.7$. In this deformation, the original global surface area has increased from 12.57 to 13.78, but the volume has decreased from 4.19 to 3.9. That means that the global area forces are trying to make the object smaller and the volume forces assigned to the same triangles are trying to make the object larger. If they are perpendicular to each other, locally this works out. However, if they are not, the in-plane portion of the volume force, depicted in Figure 3.10 (b), cancels out part of the global area force and this may cause longer relaxation times for a deformed object.

Therefore, the preferred volume forces should be perpendicular to the triangle planes.

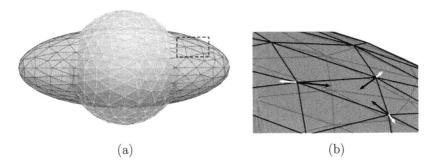

(a) (b)

FIGURE 3.10: (a) A sphere deformed into spheroid with smaller volume and larger surface. Such deformation is possible in confined geometries. (b) Smaller volume causes expanding volume forces and larger surface causes shrinking global area forces. In-plane components of volume forces (white) compete with in-plane global area forces.

3.5 Fluid-object coupling

In Section 3.1.4, we mentioned that we use two separate methods for modeling the cell and the fluid. After learning about the cell modeling part in the previous sections, we briefly get familiar with the second component in Section 3.5.1 and, more importantly, we discuss in detail the coupling between the cell model and the fluid model in Sections 3.5.2 – 3.5.5.

3.5.1 Fluid solver

The flow of the fluid, in which the cells are immersed, is usually computed from governing equations for fluid dynamics, e.g. the Navier-Stokes equations for incompressible flow [123]. Recently, the lattice-Boltzmann method (LBM) has attracted a lot of attention for its relatively simple implementation while preserving high accuracy for low and moderate Reynolds numbers [26].

This method describes the fluid dynamics and is based on fictive particles. These particles propagate and collide over a fixed three-dimensional discrete lattice. The unknown variable is the particle density function $n_i(\mathbf{x}, t)$ defined for each lattice point $\mathbf{x}$, discrete velocity vector $\mathbf{e}_i$, and time t. We use the D3Q19 version of the LBM, Figure 3.11 (three dimensions with 19 discrete directions $\mathbf{e}_i$ along the edges and diagonals of the lattice). The governing

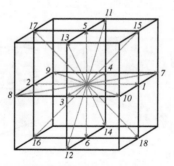

FIGURE 3.11: The D3Q19 lattice-Boltzmann directions.

equations in the presence of external forces, are

$$n_i(\mathbf{x} + \mathbf{e}_i\Delta t, t + \Delta t) = \underbrace{n_i(\mathbf{x}, t)}_{propagation} \underbrace{- \Delta_i(\mathbf{n}(\mathbf{x}, t))}_{collision} \qquad (3.10)$$

where Δt is the time step and Δ_i denotes the collision operator that accounts for the difference between pre- and post-collision states and satisfies the constraints of mass and momentum conservation. This collision operator also includes $\mathbf{F}_i$, external forces exerted on the fluid. We refer to [3] for details on the lattice-Boltzmann method. Also, a recent book [109] provides more details about principles and practice of the LBM.

The velocity field $\mathbf{u}$ and the density of the fluid ρ are evaluated from

$$\rho(\mathbf{x}, t) = \sum_i n_i(\mathbf{x}, t) \qquad \text{and} \qquad \rho(\mathbf{x}, t)\mathbf{u} = \sum_i n_i(\mathbf{x}, t)\mathbf{e}_i.$$

The cell membrane is covered by mesh points, linked together into a triangular mesh, as described before. Elastic properties of the cell membrane are represented by different force contributions corresponding to six elastic and viscous moduli. The resultant of all these forces is exerted on individual mesh points. This force causes motion of the mesh points according to Newton's equation of motion:

$$m\frac{d^2\mathbf{x}(t)}{dt^2} = \mathbf{F}_{tot}, \qquad (3.11)$$

where m is the mass of the mesh points. The sources of $\mathbf{F}_{tot}$ are either the above-mentioned elasto-mechanical properties of the cell membrane, the fluid-structure interaction or other external stimuli.

Origins of LBM method

For better understanding of the LBM, it is helpful to remember that its origins are derived from lattice gas cellular automata which is a method to simulate gas flows. The three-dimensional space is split into little cubes and gas particles travel from one such cube to another. The population of gas particles residing in one cube corresponds to local gas density and the movement of gas particles across the cube face to the neighboring cube represents gas velocity. Since liquid is *just a denser gas* (apologies for such an oversimplification), the principles of gas automata methods were taken over and the LBM has emerged.

3.5.2 Fluid-structure interaction

Equations (3.10) and (3.11) describe two different model components on two different meshes: the motion of the fluid and the motion of the immersed objects. For the coupling, we use an approach from [3, 47] based on a drag force between the fluid and the mesh points. The drag force exerted by the fluid on one mesh point is proportional to the difference of the velocity $\mathbf{v}$ of the mesh point and the fluid velocity $\mathbf{u}$ at the same position,

$$\mathbf{F} = \xi(\mathbf{u} - \mathbf{v}). \tag{3.12}$$

Here ξ is a friction coefficient.

$\mathbf{F}$ enters (3.11) as a part of $\mathbf{F}_{tot}$. The coupling is mutual so the opposite force is exerted on the fluid and $\mathbf{F}$ enters (3.10) as an external force term.

Local friction coefficient for no-slip boundary condition

The term *friction coefficient* deserves a few words. A better name would be perhaps *a no-slip coefficient* or at least *a local friction coefficient*. The current name evokes a physical resistance of relative motion of two objects or layers sliding against each other and since the object that we focus on here is a cell, it *incorrectly* evokes the resistance between the cell and the fluid. This notion is wrong because here the *friction coefficient* acts locally. It represents the physical resistance of relative motion of an individual mesh point - particle - and the fluid. While this might seem inconsequential at the first glance, it has a serious practical implication. It means that its value does not correspond to physical friction the cell experiences, but that it is a phenomenological model parameter that needs to be calibrated.

The role of the friction coefficient is to enforce the no-slip condition at the surface of the membrane. No-slip is a boundary condition used when we require fluid to be at rest at the solid boundary. Adapted for our situation, it is a condition that states that the difference of velocities of fluid and the membrane should (locally) be zero. Either the object is stationary in stationary fluid or it moves exactly with it. In the limit $\xi \to \infty$, the no-slip condition is preserved, as we see from (3.12).

In numerical computations, however, we need to use a finite value for ξ. In the next sections, the interaction between two basic parts of the model - the fluid and the cell - is properly analysed and calibrated.

This coupling is called the *force coupling algorithm* and was first introduced by Ahlrichs in [3] and later adapted by Lobaskin in [124] to model colloidal particles.

Since its inception, the force coupling algorithm has seen several improvements in terms of accuracy and flexibility. Ladd et al. [112] have devised a proper discrete integration scheme for the coupled system. A second-order accurate discretisation and a unified formalism for fluid-particle interactions including dissipative coupling, immersed boundary method and external boundary were derived by Schiller [169].

In its recent improvements [41, 64], the hydrodynamic properties of colloidal particles have been thoroughly studied. Besides spherical objects, non-spherical objects were also considered. This approach introduces a friction coefficient that needs to be properly calibrated. In the detailed analysis of the force coupling algorithm [41, 64], Fisher and coworkers examine the accuracy, with which this method is able to reproduce Stokes-level hydrodynamic interactions when compared to analytic expressions for solid spheres in simple-cubic crystals. In their work they focus on determination of the fit parameter, the effective hydrodynamic radius.

Finally, we would like to point out that the coupling done via this kind of friction coefficient makes it easy to couple the cell model to any other fluid solver, since this is the only interaction (through velocity) between the two parts of the model.

This coupling approach is termed *dissipative coupling* and since it is used to couple an immersed boundary with a fluid, we will use the abbreviation IB-DC for Immersed Boundary with Dissipative Coupling method.

Coupling via the immersed boundary method

A different approach to fluid-structure coupling is using the immersed boundary method (IBM), first introduced by Peskin [152]. For the overview of different types of IBM we refer to [132]. In IBM, the no-slip boundary condition is imposed on the membrane of the cell and the velocity of the mesh point X is set to be the velocity of the surrounding fluid $\mathbf{u}$. Because of the fixed fluid discretisation, the fluid velocity at the position $\mathbf{X}$ is obtained from convolution with a suitably chosen δ function:

$$\frac{d\mathbf{X}}{dt}(t) = \mathbf{u}(\mathbf{X}(t)) = \int \mathbf{u}(\mathbf{x})\delta(\mathbf{x} - \mathbf{X}(t))d\mathbf{x}.$$

The concrete form of the delta function influences numerical properties of the method. In [194], the authors use a smoothing technique for discrete delta function to avoid non-physical oscillations of the volume force appearing in the governing equations. In general, the choice of the proper δ function is a challenging task.

The IBM does not account for the mass of the boundary. The mesh points are massless and in situations when mass of the membrane does play a role, the use of the IBM is limited. A variant of IBM has been introduced in [105], where the authors account for the mass of the membrane by introducing a dual mesh to carry the mass. The points of the dual mesh move according to Newton's equations of motion and are linked to the original mesh by stiff springs.

An interesting connection between the dissipative coupling and immersed boundary method was pointed out by Krueger [107], where by taking the limit $\xi \to 0$ in the equations of motion in the IB-DC model with dissipative coupling, one recovers the no-slip condition on the surface and the IBM velocity interpolation.

The dissipative coupling introduces two numerical parameters ξ and m that represent the viscous friction parameter and mass of the mesh points. As discussed previously, these parameters are purely phenomenological and since the IBM does not have such parameters, it seems to be more natural. However, the time steps for the IBM and the fluid solver are required to be identical. In the approach [47], this is not the case and the *time step* for computation of spring network model can be chosen smaller than the fluid solver time step. This might be a significant advantage considering the 3D discretisation of the fluid compared to 2D membranes of the cells.

3.5.3   Computational setup

If a task is to determine the right values of a phenomenological parameter of a model, the way to do this is to test the model behavior against the expected behavior, the observed ground truth. In our case, we need to determine the value of the friction coefficient and thus the correct fluid-structure interaction. So assuming that our model of fluid-structure interaction is sound, it needs to reflect the real fluid-structure interactions.

There are numerous benchmarks for fluid-structure interaction. Most of them concern fluid dynamics around solid objects such as spheres or cylinders [119, 159]. The reason for this is that there exist analytic solutions for such simple flows.

Our aim is not the analysis of the flow profiles or velocity fields. We assume that fluid dynamics is sufficiently well governed by the lattice-Boltzmann method. Our focus is on the interaction of fluid and the object boundary and therefore we study the effects of the fluid on the object: the forces. Indeed, in our model, the function of the friction coefficient is solely the definition of forces exerted by the fluid on the object boundary.

Among the available analytic solutions to flow problems that take into account fluid forces exerted on the objects are those concerning the drag forces on an object moving in a fluid.

We have decided to set as a reference the movement of a spheroidal object (further called a sphere) in the fluid. There are theoretical computations that give us exact solutions for the velocity of such sphere. We can then compare them to computed results using our model. In this inverse way we can get the correct value for the friction coefficient.

The motion of solid objects immersed in fluid is described by Newton's second law of motion:

$$\mathbf{F} = m\frac{d\mathbf{v}}{dt}, \tag{3.13}$$

where m is mass and $\mathbf{v}$ is the velocity of the object. We focus on flow with low Reynolds number and for these, the drag force of the fluid on the objects is given by Stokes law as

$$\mathbf{F}_d = 6\pi\mu r\mathbf{v}, \tag{3.14}$$

where r is radius of the object, $\mathbf{v}$ is its velocity relative to the surrounding fluid and μ is dynamic viscosity of the fluid. The theory assumes a solid rigid object immersed in an unbounded fluid. Our model assumes elastic objects. By setting the elastic coefficients high enough we can achieve that reasonably well with our model.

Then there is of course the question of the *unbounded domain*. There is a suggested aspect ratio between the size of the sphere and the computational domain that must be used in order to avoid boundary effects. Authors in [21] discuss this issue and the ratio 1:20 seems to be sufficient. With the sphere diameter $10\mu m$ and the simulation box of dimensions $200 \times 200 \times 200\mu m^3$, the relative error of the velocity field in each point of space was below 5%. We consider such accuracy sufficient in view of the fact that in other works, e.g. [107], a smaller simulation box (relatively to the object size) was used in a similar scenario.

In the following, we describe two similar experiments.

Terminal velocity experiment

We put a sphere into a static fluid. Constant horizontal force $\mathbf{F}_0$ is applied on the sphere, see Figure 3.12 (a). The sphere accelerates and the drag force increases as a result. At some point it cancels out with $\mathbf{F}_0$, and the sphere velocity stabilises at some value. We call this value *terminal velocity* and denote it by $\mathbf{v}_\infty$. The terminal velocity can be derived from theoretical assumptions similarly as in [21]. We calculate terminal velocity by the following formula:

$$\mathbf{v}_\infty = \lim_{t\to\infty} \mathbf{v}(t) = \frac{\mathbf{F}_0}{6\pi\mu r}. \tag{3.15}$$

The terminal velocity does not depend on the object mass.

Balancing force experiment

We put a sphere into a fluid flowing with constant velocity $\mathbf{v}_0$. We exert a horizontal *balancing force* denoted by $\mathbf{F}_A$ in the direction opposite to the flow such that the sphere remains stationary, see Figure 3.12 (b). According to

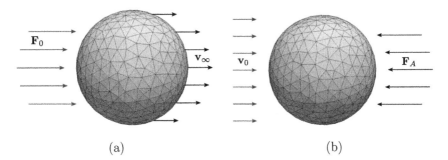

(a)   (b)

FIGURE 3.12: (a) Terminal velocity experiment, where force is initialised to $\mathbf{F}_0$ and terminal velocity $\mathbf{v}_\infty$ is simulated. (b) Balancing force experiment, where velocity of fluid is initialised to $\mathbf{v}_0$ and adaptive force $\mathbf{F}_A$ is simulated.

the theory, the balancing force exerted on the sphere in an equilibrium state equals the drag force given by Stokes law. We calculate the exact expression by the following formula:

$$\mathbf{F}_A = 6\pi\mu r \mathbf{v}_0. \qquad (3.16)$$

Again, this does not depend on the object mass.

3.5.4 Identification of the friction coefficient

We identify the friction coefficient gradually in four stages:

- Friction calibration for a reference sphere

- Generalisation to an arbitrary sphere

- Generalisation to an arbitrary shape

- Validation for ellipsoidal shapes

First, we calibrate the friction coefficient for one specific sphere and denote it *reference sphere*. Then we derive a formula for general sphere involving the radius and number of mesh points defining the dependence of friction coefficient on those two parameters. Finally, we generalise the result for an arbitrary shape using the density of the mesh. This result will be tested using the available benchmark - the explicit formulas for drag force of rotational ellipsoids.

Friction calibration for a reference sphere

First, we perform a computer simulation of both experiments. We pick an initial value of ξ and we check whether the simulated values of terminal velocity in the first experiment and balancing force in the second experiment correspond to the theoretical values. If not (which is highly probable for the first shot), we adapt the value of ξ and try again. By this inverse process we are able to determine the correct value of ξ. We use the simple bisection/step doubling method.

Computationally, this process is quite demanding. To evaluate both experiments for one single value of ξ we need to perform a full 3D simulation. The iteration process of finding the correct value involves tens of such steps. So it is not such a good idea to perform this process for each new mesh. Therefore, we first calibrate ξ_{ref} for one reference sphere and afterwards we derive a formula for direct computation of ξ for an arbitrary sphere based on the value ξ_{ref}.

Since the red blood cell has a radius approximately $4\,\mu m$, we pick a sphere with this radius 4 as the reference sphere. The reference number of mesh points was chosen to be 393.

The remaining simulation parameters together with the detailed results are presented in [21]. The observed behavior was as expected: In the case of the terminal velocity experiment, increasing the friction causes a decrease in the terminal velocity. This is natural, since increasing the friction coefficient means that the effect of fluid on the object is stronger and thus it slows the sphere down more for larger values of ξ. The value, for which the simulated terminal velocity matched the expected theoretical velocity computed from (3.15), was $1.82nNs/m$.

In case of the balancing force experiment, increasing the friction means that the fluid acts on the object stronger and thus we need a larger balancing force to keep the object in place. The value of ξ, for which the balancing force matched the theoretical value from (3.16), was the same as in the previous case.

Together, the experiments have determined the calibrated value of the friction coefficient for the reference sphere as

$$\xi_{ref} = 1.82nNs/m.$$

Generalisation for an arbitrary sphere

To determine the influence of the number of nodes n and radius r of sphere mesh, let us do some brainstorming about the terminal velocity experiment.

Friction coefficients for meshes with different densities and sizes
First, we analyse the situation for two different meshes with number of mesh points n_1 and n_2 and the radius of the sphere fixed. We want to find out the relation between the corresponding friction coefficients ξ_1 and ξ_2 in order to achieve the same simulated behavior.

As soon as the sphere reaches the terminal velocity, all forces exerted on the mesh points come to an equilibrium. There are three types of forces exerted on the mesh points: elastic forces, external force $\mathbf{F}_0$ that pulls the object and fluid forces that act in the direction opposite to $\mathbf{F}_0$. The elastic forces just keep the sphere almost solid and do not contribute to the balance between the external force and the fluid force. So basically, in each mesh point we have the equilibrium of the external force and the fluid force. We can use (3.12) to calculate the fluid force and thus for both meshes we have

$$\mathbf{F}_0 = \sum_{i=1}^{n_1} \xi_1(\mathbf{u}_i - \mathbf{v}_i) = \sum_{i=1}^{n_2} \xi_2(\mathbf{u}_i - \mathbf{v}_i).$$

Our aim is to get the same behavior of the simulated sphere in the computational experiment and thus the velocities $\mathbf{u}_i$ of mesh points for both meshes will be the same. The same holds for the fluid interpolated velocities $\mathbf{v}_i$ and thus we can conclude that

$$\sum_{i=1}^{n_1} \xi_1 = \sum_{i=1}^{n_2} \xi_2 \quad \text{or} \quad n_1 \xi_1 = n_2 \xi_2. \tag{3.17}$$

Second, we analyse the situation when we keep the number of mesh points fixed, equal to n and we have two different radii r_1 and r_2. Assume that we want to use two different dragging forces $\mathbf{F}_1$ and $\mathbf{F}_2$ to get the same terminal velocity for both spheres. In the equilibrium, the dragging forces $\mathbf{F}_1, \mathbf{F}_2$ are compensated by the drag force computed from (3.14) and thus we get

$$\mathbf{F}_1 = 6\pi\mu r_1 \mathbf{v}_\infty = \sum_{i=1}^{n} \xi_1(\mathbf{u}_i - \mathbf{v}_i)$$

$$\mathbf{F}_2 = 6\pi\mu r_2 \mathbf{v}_\infty = \sum_{i=1}^{n} \xi_2(\mathbf{u}_i - \mathbf{v}_i)$$

With similar reasoning as before we note that both spheres are moving with the same terminal velocity and thus $\mathbf{u}_i$ and $\mathbf{v}_i$ are the same. Using this result, after dividing the previous two equations we end up with

$$\frac{r_1}{r_2} = \frac{\xi_1}{\xi_2} \tag{3.18}$$

To derive an explicit formula describing the dependence of the friction coefficient on the parameters of the sphere mesh, we can now use formulas (3.17) and (3.18). Plainly, the relations say that

the friction coefficient increases linearly with
the increasing radius of the sphere

and

> *the friction coefficient decreases linearly with*
> *the increasing number of nodes*

This can be summarised in the following formula:

$$\xi_{n,r} = \frac{n_{ref}}{n}\frac{r}{r_{ref}}\xi_{ref}. \tag{3.19}$$

To validate the previous relation, we have performed a number of simulations varying the radius of the sphere and the number of mesh points. The details are provided in [21]. We have compared the simulated terminal velocity using the friction coefficient prescribed by (3.19) and the expected terminal velocity computed using the theoretical equation (3.15). In all the simulations, the relative error was below 5%.

Generalisation for an arbitrary shape

Now that we know how to compute the friction coefficient for a spherical object, the question remains: What is the correct friction coefficient for non-spherical objects? The general function of the friction coefficient is to transfer the drag force of the fluid onto the object and back. Since the object is modeled by its membrane only, we need to transfer this drag force solely by the mesh points. Naturally, for a denser mesh, it is sufficient to transfer less force per mesh node to get the same effect on the membrane. It is thus logical to expect that the friction coefficient depends inversely on the *density* of the mesh points. This idea is supported by the expression (3.19): Increasing the number of mesh points while preserving the radius increases the *density* of mesh points and decreases the value of ξ.

Next, we need to define the mesh *density*. The first approximation could be the number of mesh points per unit area, explicitly expressed by n/S, where S is the surface of the object. However, the relation (3.19) suggests something different: It defines the mesh *density* as the number of mesh points per a unit length. In case of spheres, the *density* could be defined as n/r. For general shapes, we could replace the radius with one half of the maximal diameter of the object (think sphere vs. frisbee).

The problem is that this would not reflect the fact that keeping the diameter and number of mesh points constant, one can increase the surface, which subsequently decreases the mesh *density*. Therefore, we suggest using the square root of the surface. For spheres, this choice is equivalent (up to a multiplicative constant) with using the radius. Our proposition is to use the following expression for the computation of the friction coefficient for non-spherical objects with n mesh points and surface S:

$$\xi_{n,S} = \frac{n_{ref}}{n}\frac{\sqrt{S}}{\sqrt{S_{ref}}}\xi_{ref}. \tag{3.20}$$

Note, that for spheres, the newly proposed relation is consistent with (3.19). The formula is now shape independent.

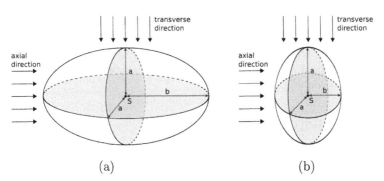

FIGURE 3.13: Ellipsoids and their axial and transverse directions. (a) Prolate ellipsoid with circular cross section with diameter a and prolonged radius b. (b) Oblate ellipsoid with circular cross section with diameter a and shortened radius b.

Validation for ellipsoidal shapes

To verify the hypotheses we use theoretical results concerning movement of rotationally symmetric ellipsoids in a fluid. Such ellipsoids are created from a sphere by prolonging (prolate ellipsoids) or shortening (oblate ellipsoids) the sphere along one axis, see Figure 3.13. The modified radius is denoted by b.

The relation (3.14) that is valid for spherical objects can be generalised for oblate and prolate ellipsoids [30]. The explicit expression for the drag force reads as

$$\mathbf{F}_d = 6\pi\mu aK\mathbf{v}, \tag{3.21}$$

where μ is the dynamic viscosity of the fluid, $\mathbf{v}$ is the relative velocity of the ellipsoid to the fluid, a is the radius of circular cross section of the ellipsoid and K is a shape factor. K depends on the ratio a/b and on the flow direction. The concrete values of K for different cases can be found in [23, 30].

Using (3.21) we can repeat the theoretical steps from the previous sections and conclude that $\mathbf{v}_\infty$ for the terminal velocity experiment and $\mathbf{F}_A$ for the balancing force experiment read as

$$\mathbf{v}_\infty = \frac{\mathbf{F}_0}{6\pi\mu aK} \quad \text{and} \quad \mathbf{F}_A = 6\pi\mu aK\mathbf{v}_0.$$

These expressions give us the expected values of $\mathbf{v}_\infty$ and $\mathbf{F}_A$ in both experiments.

To test our hypothesis (3.20), we have chosen six different ellipsoids (three of them were prolate and three were oblate). Each ellipsoid was triangulated using open-source software Gmsh [74]. The triangulation was regular and thus the local density of mesh points was approximately constant across the surface of the ellipsoid. The dimensions and other information are available in [23].

As in the case of spherical objects, we have compared the simulated terminal velocity (and balancing force) using the friction coefficient prescribed by (3.19) and the expected terminal velocity (and balancing force) computed from the theoretical equation (3.15). In all simulations, we have obtained a relative error below 5%.

3.5.5   Sensitivity analysis

Next we analyse how sensitive is the derived formula on other simulation parameters. Besides the friction, we have the following:

- *Model parameters:* Size of simulation box, elastic coefficients of the sphere, time step, fluid grid size, mass of mesh points

- *Parameters of control experiments:* Dragging force $\mathbf{F}_0$, fluid velocity $\mathbf{v}_0$

- *Physical properties:* Viscosity, density

In the following, we check whether perturbations in these parameters have influence on the computed value of the friction coefficient. A series of simulations can be performed for each parameter in the list above, varying its value and keeping other parameters fixed.

Let us discuss the first group of parameters. The influence of the size of the simulation box has already been analysed in [21]. The conclusions are that setting the size of the simulation box to at least $200\mu m$ is sufficient to eliminate the artificial boundary influence on the results. The elastic coefficients are taken high enough to keep the deformation of the sphere negligible and they do not influence the results, when the sphere does not deform.

The size of the time step naturally influences the accuracy of the time derivative approximation, but this is not linked to the friction coefficient.

When a fluid is modeled, an important parameter is size of its discretisation. In the lattice-Boltzmann method the fluid is computed on a cubic lattice with a given grid size that is the same in all three spatial directions. So far, in all friction calibration simulations we have used grid size $1\mu m$. A series of simulations with different values of the grid size had shown no influence of the grid size on the results.

The last parameter from this group is the mass of the particles. The mass parameter in our model is not a mass of the modeled object in a physical meaning. From the simulation experience, we can say that the particles forming the mesh oscillate around an equilibrium state on much smaller time and space scales than the deformations and movements of the object. The particle mass only influences the speed and the magnitude of these fast and small oscillations. However, if the numerical computation remains stable, the modeled object behaves the same way even with changing mass of the particles. This has been demonstrated by a series of simulations with varying mass of particles indicating no influence on the friction coefficient.

The second group contains parameters of the experiments: the dragging force F_0 and the fluid velocity v_0. These parameters are not linked to the physical properties and thus we expect that the calibrated friction is independent of these parameters. Results from series of experiments with varying these parameters have revealed no influence on the resulting friction coefficient.

The last group of parameters contains physical properties of the fluid. Here, we can expect some dependence of the calibrated friction since the friction coefficient is responsible for transfer of forces between the fluid and immersed objects. If the fluid has a larger viscosity, it naturally affects the immersed objects more. Our preliminary simulations have shown that indeed the friction coefficient for the reference sphere is different for various viscosities. Therefore, we have performed the calibration of a reference sphere for three typical fluids used in microfluidics.

A natural first choice is blood plasma. The values of blood plasma viscosity vary from 1.3 to $1.5mPa.s$ [86, 104]. The other two fluids are phosphate-buffered saline suspensions used, e.g. in [40, 136]. All three fluids have the same density $1025kg.m^{-3}$ and their respective viscosities are presented in Table 3.4. It shows the calibrated friction coefficient for the reference sphere with 393 nodes and radius 4 μm. The relation (3.20) remains valid, with different values for the reference sphere.

$\mu\ [mPa\,s]$	$\xi\ [nN\,s\,m^{-1}]$
1.5375	1.82
1.3000	1.54
1.0000	1.18

TABLE 3.4: Calibrated friction coefficient for the reference sphere for three different fluids, from [23].

3.5.6   Flow through membrane

Every choice has a price. Sometimes we do not know what it is until we have paid it. Once we choose to use a spring network model with particles on the surface of the membrane and dissipative coupling of these particles with fluid, we pay the price of fluid flowing through the membrane. We need to be aware of this kind of imperfections of our models and wherever we can, we should also quantify them. Find out what the price was at least after you have paid it. Ideally, we should know or decide in advance what the acceptable error (price) is.

The assumption is that a no-slip condition should hold on the cell surface and the inner volume should be conserved at all times. This is expected biologically, since under constant osmotic conditions, the changes in cell volume are negligible. On the other hand, if the no-slip condition does not hold, there is a non-zero velocity difference between fluid velocity and cell velocity at the boundary and thus a non-zero flux through the membrane.

The non-zero velocity difference is what drives the dissipative coupling as described in Section 3.5.2, therefore the goal is not to eliminate it altogether, but rather to quantify the effect and confirm that it is negligible with respect to other dynamics of the cell. The adjective *dissipative* refers to the fact that we do not have a discontinuity in velocity at the surface of the cell, but rather use interpolated velocities from nearby lattice nodes and thus introduce interpolation errors that dissipate away in both directions from the boundary.

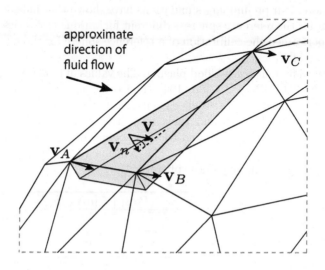

FIGURE 3.14: Flow through one face of the membrane.

We can estimate the flow through the membrane in one time step by the following method. We run a cycle over the surface triangles. For each triangle we calculate the differences of the velocity of triangle nodes and interpolated fluid velocity at the same positions. We denote these differences for one particular triangle depicted in Figure 3.14 by $\mathbf{v}_A, \mathbf{v}_B, \mathbf{v}_C$. Only these differences enter the calculation of flow through the membrane because if both the membrane and the surrounding fluid moved with the same velocity (and thus had a zero velocity difference) there would be no leak through the membrane.

We take the average of the three velocity difference vectors to obtain the velocity difference per triangle $\mathbf{v} = 1/3(\mathbf{v}_A + \mathbf{v}_B + \mathbf{v}_C)$ and then we calculate the projection $\mathbf{v}_n$ of the resulting velocity vector $\mathbf{v}$ on the triangle normal $\mathbf{n}$ using the formula

$$\mathbf{v}_n = \frac{(\mathbf{v}, \mathbf{n})}{(\mathbf{n}, \mathbf{n})}\mathbf{n}.$$

We do this projection because the vector can be decomposed into the normal and tangential component, but only the normal component represents the flow through the membrane.

Next, we compute the volume of the fluid by multiplying the norm of the projection by the triangle area, see Figure 3.14, and finally add the result to the total sum of all partial volume contributions. This method is also written in the following code snippet and outputs the leak through the membrane in one time step as a percentage of the total cell volume:

```
# calculation of flow through a membrane
flow_through_membrane = 0
for t in cell.mesh.triangles:
    posA = t.A.get_pos()
    posB = t.B.get_pos()
    posC = t.C.get_pos()
    velDiffA = t.A.get_vel() - lbf.get_interpolated_velocity(posA)
    velDiffB = t.B.get_vel() - lbf.get_interpolated_velocity(posB)
    velDiffC = t.C.get_vel() - lbf.get_interpolated_velocity(posC)
    avg_vel = np.array(velDiffA + velDiffB + velDiffC)/3.0
    normal = np.array(oif.get_triangle_normal(posA, posB, posC))
    proj_avg_vel = (np.inner(avg_vel, normal)/np.inner(normal, normal)) \
    * normal
    size_proj_avg_vel = oif.norm(proj_avg_vel)
    partial_volume = size_proj_avg_vel * \
    oif.area_triangle(posA, posB, posC)
    flow_through_membrane = flow_through_membrane + partial_volume
print "flow through membrane in percent of volume: ", \
str(flow_through_membrane/cell.volume()*100)
```

If instead by volume, we divide the total flow through the membrane by the cell surface, we obtain a numerical approximation of the physical quantity called volumetric flow, which is a flow rate per unit area. The rate in this definition means that the calculation is done per time step. This could be useful for comparing flows through various membranes.

To calculate the fluid velocity at the position of the membrane node we have to use 3D interpolation, such as that depicted in Figure 3.15. To calculate the velocity at membrane node M, we weigh the velocities in lattice nodes $L_1, \ldots, L_8$ in such a way that velocity in L_1 is weighted by the volume of the box with the opposite corner L_7, etc. This is called trilinear interpolation.

Note that the flow through the membrane is not unique to the IB-DC model. Also in IBM+LBM models, such as [107], the no-slip condition on the surface of the membrane is not satisfied exactly - for two reasons. One is that fluid in LBM is incompressible in the hydrodynamic limit only. And the second is that the interpolated velocity field is not generally divergence-free. This leads to the introduction of phenomenological membrane volume energetics, i.e. volume modulus, that compensates for the flow through the membrane and keeps it under a predefined amount.

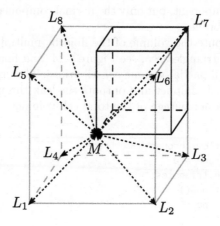

FIGURE 3.15: Trilinear velocity interpolation.

Things to ponder

How does the flow through the membrane change with increasing velocity of the fluid?

How does the flow through the membrane change when we change the orientation of the red blood cell with respect to the flow direction?

What is the flow through the membrane of the red blood cell when the cell is being squeezed between two obstacles?

3.6 Cell-cell interaction

Blood is a dense fluid. To get an idea just how dense, consider this: blood cells occupy roughly half of the total blood volume. At first, this might not sound especially *full*, but once we take into account the shape of the cells, with their two concavities, and consider the fact that the cells are not neatly arranged, suddenly the 50% volume fraction results in a seriously overcrowded space. For comparison, in the densest sphere packing, the spheres occupy around 74% of the total volume - this is in case all the spheres are the same size. In case they are not, random sphere packings generally give densities around 64% [177].

In these dense settings, the cell-cell interactions happen frequently, and it is necessary to consider them carefully. In experimental settings, the cell-cell interactions have been observed on a larger scale quite some time ago: for RBCs [17]. However, only recently the study of relatively controlled pairings of two cells have become possible: for lymphocytes [49], for RBCs in shear flow [144].

There are two basic theories that describe them: bridging between cells by cross-linking molecules [28], and the balance of osmotic forces generated by the depletion of molecules in the intercellular space [139]. Both of them assume that the membranes attract each other when the surfaces are close enough and then they repel each other, if they come too close. A review of deformation and interaction models of RBCs can be found in [103].

Membrane self-repulsion to prevent mesh self-overlapping

When an extreme deformation of a cell occurs in biological flow, one part of the cell membrane may be forced to touch another part of the same cell membrane. This may happen when a cell is deformed e.g. into a C-shape. In that case, two parts of the same membrane may approach each other and their outer sides may touch.

In our cell model, the mesh of one cell can in principle self-overlap. To prevent this, a repulsive mechanism may be added so that the particles of a mesh repel each other when reaching a critical cutoff distance. Such a mechanism may be implemented with a non-bonded potential, similarly to the repulsive cell-cell interactions discussed later in this section.

How do we account for this behavior in the model? A collision detection algorithm should be run between all appropriate pairs of objects and suitable response performed when they are close enough.

Collision detection algorithms have been extensively explored and applied in computer games, animation, physics-based modeling, molecular modeling, robot motion planning, virtual reality, etc. [120]. The most common approach is to enclose each object in a bounding volume (box, sphere or other) and at first only check whether these volumes came into contact. The reasoning behind this approach is that a computationally inexpensive check can be done often to exclude pairs that definitely could not have intersected. Such a check means comparing the distance of centers with the sum of two radii in case of spheres or mutual position of opposite bounding box corners in case of boxes.

Only those pairs that possibly could have come into contact, meaning that the encapsulated objects are sufficiently close, are then examined more carefully - the actual boundaries of the objects are used to check whether the collision has truly happened.

A side note: the collision detection theory distinguishes between *a priori* detection and *a posteriori* detection. The *a priori* detection catches situations when the objects might collide by predicting their near future trajectories and the *a posteriori* detection typically misses the actual collision and reacts only after it has already happened. As we will see later, in models of elastic objects, it is possible to do a somewhat strange mix of these two approaches:

repulsive forces are applied before the collision happens and in case these are not sufficient, a correction mechanism is employed after the collision.

A natural approach in the spring network models is to transform the object-object interaction into a set of particle-particle interactions. The pairs of particles then receive repulsive forces when they get too close. The forces correspond to the *soft-sphere potential*:

$$V(d) = ad^{-n}, \qquad d < d_{cut}, \tag{3.22}$$

where d is the distance between the two particles, d_{cut} is the threshold at which this potential starts acting (for larger distances, no force is applied to these two particles), a is a scaling parameter and n (typically greater than 1) determines how *steep* the response gets as particles approach one another. Unlike the elastic interactions, this interaction only works when two points of predefined types - any two points of predefined types - get sufficiently close. How close is sufficiently close? Closer than d_{cut}. This is the reason why this type of interaction is typically called non-bonded.

In practice this means that particles of one object are of one type. Particles of another object are of a second type. Recall that we have seen these particle types in the example in Chapter 2. Some of them enter the interaction because the objects got close enough. And the collective effect of interactions between the two groups of particles is that the two objects repel each other when they are on a collision course. The drawback of this approach is that in the event that the two objects intersect, instead of correcting this unphysical behavior and pushing them apart, this type of potential locks them in even more. An illustration of this effect can be seen in Figure 3.16 (a).

How is it possible that they intersect? Obviously the biological cells do not get into each other's personal space and therefore neither should the simulated cells. This is of course a sound requirement, but practically, in dense simulations, it is difficult to achieve without applying too strong a repulsive potential that results in a protective boundary layer around the cell most of the time.

Due to a numerical integration step, a particle mesh point of one object may *cross* the membrane of the neighboring object sooner than the repulsive potential has had a chance to deflect its trajectory. The soft-sphere potential should repulse the two membranes, but this time the repulsion means that the membranes intersect even further. One way to remedy this problem is to decrease the time step, so that the repulsion has time to react. As an alternative, the following collision algorithm can be used.

It takes into account not only the distance of the two points but also the normal vectors of the two corresponding objects at these two points. Based on these two vectors, it determines whether the two membranes have crossed each other or not and applies the repulsive forces in the proper direction, Figure 3.16.

This approach requires a different distance-dependent potential, since we now need it inversely proportional to the distance of nodes of membranes

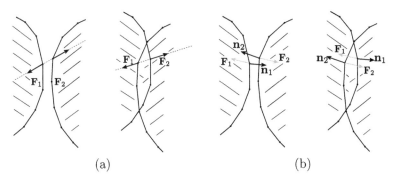

(a)   (b)

FIGURE 3.16: 2D illustration and comparison of two types of repulsion.
(a) Soft-sphere repulsive potential - regardless of the relative positions of the
two membranes, opposite forces $\mathbf{F}_1$ and $\mathbf{F}_2$ are added to each pair of affected
nodes along the dashed line joining them. (b) Membrane collision repulsive
potential - determination of force direction depends on the outward normals
$\mathbf{n}_1$ and $\mathbf{n}_2$ of the two affected nodes.

that are not crossed and saturating with growing distance of nodes of crossed
membranes, as depicted in Figure 3.17. One example of such potential is

$$V(d) = a\frac{1}{1 + e^{nd}} \qquad d < d_{cut}, \tag{3.23}$$

where d is the distance between the two particles, d_{cut} is the threshold, at
which this potential starts acting (for larger distances, no force is applied to
these two particles), a is a scaling parameter and n (typically greater than 1)
determines how *steep* the response gets as particles approach one another. Of
course, other potentials that have the same property could be used.

The collision detection algorithm then works as follows: It detects the
proximity of two points of different types and applies repulsive potential in
the direction $\mathbf{dir} = \mathbf{n}_{P1} - \mathbf{n}_{P2}$.

```
# membrane collision interaction
If dist(P1, P2) < dist_cut:
        F_P1 = V(dist) * dir
        F_P2 = -V(dist) * dir
```

This method depends on a straightforward calculation of the (at least
approximate) outward normal vector at any given mesh node at any given
time, Figure 3.18, since the membranes are moving both due to the advection
and due to elastic deformations. The mesh, however, is a polygonal object,
for which it is impossible to define an outward normal vector at its vertex.
Therefore, we work with an approximation. One possible way to calculate the
approximation of outward normal is as follows.

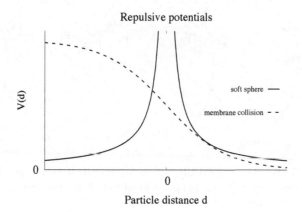

FIGURE 3.17: Two types of object-object repulsive potentials.

During the initialisation phase, we identify all neighbors of each node. Since the mesh connectivity remains the same during the whole simulation, the neighbors do not change either. For each node P, we select three of its neighbors N_1, N_2, N_3 that are best spatially distributed, by checking all triplets of neighbors and choosing the one, for which the following expression is minimal:

$$\min_{i,j,k} |(\mathbf{N}_i - \mathbf{P}) + (\mathbf{N}_j - \mathbf{P}) + (\mathbf{N}_k - \mathbf{P})|,$$

where $N_i, N_j, N_k \in S$ and S is the set of all neighbors of mesh node P. This expression would be 0 if P was the centroid of an equilateral triangle $N_iN_jN_k$. The maximum value is reached when PN_iN_j and PN_jN_k are adjacent triangles.

A typical node has six or seven neighbors, which means about $\binom{7}{3} = 35$ checks per node. In ESPResSo, these checks are done only once for each cell type, because the identified neighbors can be used in all cells created based on the given type.

Once the neighbors are identified, we compute the normal $\mathbf{n}_P$ of the triangle $N_1N_2N_3$. This normal may point inside or outside of the object, depending on the order of nodes N_i. By checking the angle between $\mathbf{n}_P$ and the normal of any mesh triangle containing node P, we determine the proper orientation and reorder the nodes $N_1N_2N_3$, if necessary, so that the normal of a triangle with reordered nodes points outward. The IDs of these three nodes in proper order are then saved in the particle structure of node P and anytime during the simulation when outward normal at P is necessary, it is computed from their current positions as any other bonded interaction.

With this algorithm in place, we no longer see entangled membranes.

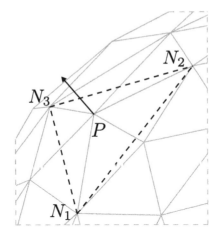

FIGURE 3.18: Outward normal for a given mesh node.

Algorithm for initialisation of membrane collision
In order for the membrane collision to work properly, we need to set up a bonded interaction when the object is created. The steps are as follows:

- Identify all neighbors of a given node. These do not change during simulation.

- Select the three neighbors that are best spatially distributed.

- Compute the normal of the triangle defined by the three selected neighbors.

- Determine the outward direction of this normal with respect to the object.

- Save these three nodes in the correct order to have the proper orientation of the triangle determined by them.

- Use these three nodes to compute the normal of the given node any time during the simulation.

Returning briefly to our earlier discussion of force-free and torque-free forces, we should also consider the cell-cell interaction from this angle. Clearly, it is force-free when considering the two objects as one system, since the force of the same magnitude with opposite direction is applied to a pair of mesh points. The direction of this force is in general different than the direction of the line connecting the two mesh points and therefore this kind of interaction is not torque free. It is neither force- nor torque-free with respect to a single object, but we cannot expect that for any kind of cell-cell interaction.

3.7   Brief overview of other approaches

In simulations of RBC flows, the length scale is usually about several micrometers to several hundreds of micrometers. This means we are looking for methods that have the resolution capable of looking at individual cell deformations and at the same time include several (the more, the better) cells.

3.7.1   Categorisation of red cell models

These methods fall into two basic categories: continuum models, in which the membrane properties are described by equations and network-based models, in which the interactions of network nodes give rise to membrane properties. The network resolution ranges from very fine, at the level of atomistic simulations, to quite coarse, such as in [147], where 10 colloidal particles are arranged into a closed torus-like ring and by worm-like chain (WLC) springs combined with bending resistance. The fact that this approach is based on the structural biochemical design of the cells also makes it the reasonable starting point in applications that concern various diseases, such as sickle cell anemia, malaria, etc., which affect the function of the structure.

Continuum models

Continuum models treat the membrane as a thin shell and track its deformations in time [80, 157]. The great advantage of these models is that they can be treated with a large number of well-developed numerical techniques.

When considering just the membrane shear modulus, the solutions can be found analytically, but once another material parameter is added, i.e. the bending modulus, computer simulations are needed to get the results. This is a stiff problem, since the contribution of the bending modulus to the uniaxial deformation is much smaller than the contribution from the shear modulus [131]. Modelers also need to keep in mind the large deformations that red blood cells undergo. This issue may be overcome by mesh-free methods, such as in [123], but the general preference in blood cell modeling on a single-cell level seems to lean more towards the network-based models.

Atomistic simulations of lipid bilayers

The fine network-based models look in detail at the membrane as a lipid bilayer with the underlaying spectrin filament network [116, 118, 164]. In principle, all individual atoms could be included, but in practice, this would not be reasonable. Typically, multiple atoms are clustered together. Using this kind of model, it is also possible to recover the thermal fluctuations of the membrane and examine how the lipid bilayer and spectrin filaments affect each other. For a review of the molecular dynamics simulations of lipid bilayers see [61].

Thermal fluctuations

Thermal fluctuations are random deviations of a system - in our context a membrane - from its equilibrium value. The word *thermal* refers to statistical mechanics, where at any temperature larger than absolute zero, the atoms move around. The higher the temperature is, the larger and more frequent the movement.

For our membrane this means that while we have a biconcave discoid representation of the relaxed membrane shape, in reality, the membrane surface constantly undergoes *zig-zag* oscillations *around* this biconcave discoid equilibrium. The amplitudes of the fluctuations are at the scale of tens to lower hundreds *nm* and beyond the resolution of the model presented in this work. An example of an RBC model that includes the thermal fluctuations can be found in [126].

Particle-based models

In some network-based models, not only are the network nodes particles, but the physical fluid is also clustered into similar particles, such as in Dissipative Particle Dynamics (DPD) [56, 155]. This notion is called coarse-graining and allows the use of the same model for a cell discretised with 100 nodes, which is around the minimum necessary to have the proper RBC shape and be able to observe deformations, and for a cell discretised with 27,000 nodes, which is about the number of spectrin filament crossings in the membrane. Macroscopic quantities, such as velocity and density, are reconstructed from the positions and velocities of the particles. Different types of particles are used to distinguish between the inside of the cell, its membrane, outer fluid and walls. All are governed by conservative, dissipative and stochastic forces but in addition to that, the membrane particles form a network of elastic or viscoelastic springs.

The great flexibility of this stochastic method, the fact that the cell-fluid interaction does not need special treatment, since it is a particle-particle interaction like any other and the ability to easily coarse-grain comes at a price that the physical constants have to be accounted for very carefully in the conservative and dissipative forces - it is problematic to change one parameter independently of the others. Also, there are no clear physical scales, since the forces are not derived from a physical model, and it is necessary to make assumptions about the mass of the membrane particles (typically different from the mass of the cytoplasm particle).

Some of the drawbacks of DPD are taken care of in the Smoothed Particle Hydrodynamics (SPH) method, which is more of a macroscopic method. The force formulation is similar as in DPD, but the SPH forces are derived from Navier-Stokes equations and thus the physical density and velocity can be obtained directly [97]. It is problematic to account for the viscoelastic behavior of the membrane and the concerns about the specification of mass of membrane particles remain.

Multiparticle collision dynamics is another mesoscopic model for the solvent [78]. Coupled with a dynamically triangulated surface model for the membrane [142] it can also recover thermal fluctuations of the solvent and of the membrane.

For a more detailed comparison of particle-based models, see [195].

Mesh-based models

Mesh-based models study the biomechanical properties of the cell membrane by looking at a similar triangular network as particle-based models with fixed connectivity of mesh nodes. Typically, this mesh is coupled to a lattice-Boltzmann (LBM) representation of the fluid [200], which uses a cubic lattice. The advantage is that the fluid dynamics is local and thus very suitable for parallelisation.

The cell-fluid coupling may be done via the immersed boundary method (IBM) developed in [153], such as in [107] or using a dissipative coupling, as described in Section 3.5. While both approaches obey momentum conservation, the straightforward dissipative coupling introduces an additional unphysical parameter that needs to be set.

The RBC elasticity may be specified either using forces, e.g. in Chapter 3 or [40], or energetic description, e.g. [189]. In some cases, both approaches lead to an identical implementation of elastic moduli.

With these methods, it is necessary to keep in mind that the average edge length in the cell mesh should be about Δx (spatial discretisation step) with small variance. If it is significantly smaller, the interpolation of velocity of the nodes from the velocity of the surrounding fluid gives very similar results. Since apart from viscoelasticity this is the only information that is used to propagate the nodes, they thus move with almost the same velocity. This may lead to membranes *sticking together* [107].

3.7.2 Comparison of models and solvers

In Chapter 4 we discuss how a model can be compared to biological reality, but before we get there, it is worth looking at how a model can be compared to other models. This is a useful exploration, since no single method can be expected to be universally advantageous. Different applications call for strengths of different methods.

We have denoted the model introduced in this chapter by IB-DC (Immersed Boundary via Dissipative Coupling). More precisely, it should be IB-DC+LBM, but we omit the LBM for simplicity. Consider now, how it fits among some other mesoscopic models, namely the DPD model [56] and the IBM+LBM model [107] (in the following text just IBM, for shorter notation).

While the fluid-object interaction is different in each of these three models, one thing they have in common is the triangular mesh representing the object and definition of forces/energies that define the elastic behavior.

First some general remarks on the cell flow properties that the models try to capture:

- **Cell-fluid interaction:** Compared to DPD and IB-DC, the cell-fluid interaction is more physical in the IBM model. In DPD, the RBC membrane consists of the same kind of particles as the fluid and cell-fluid interactions are treated directly as particle-particle interactions. This approach is straightforward and simple, but the drawback is that the RBC membrane needs to have a negligible mass compared with the mass of the inner cytoplasm. If a large number of particles are used to model the membrane, their combined masses should be far less than the mass of cytoplasm, which leads to a small time step. IBM does not face this issue and enforces a no-slip condition on the membrane boundary using the discretised delta functions without any artificial parameters. While IB-DC also uses velocity interpolation from the underlying fluid lattice and subsequent force spreading, the spring network nodes have mass too, which enters Newton's equation of motion. This means they are subject to similar restrictions as DPD.

- **Cell-cell and cell-wall interactions:** It is well known that the fluid models are not accurate in narrow gaps - if the distance between two objects becomes less than the spatial step. This distance is much larger than the distance between biological red blood cells at high volume fractions ($\sim 13nm$ [195]). In all three considered mesoscale models, this leads to issues with both cell-cell interactions and cell-wall interactions, because they are not capable of resolving the small separation. All of them need to make sure that the cell maintains a minimum distance from the walls. This means that the behavior close to the walls is unphysical because they employ cell-cell repulsive forces [63, 107]. In general, the goal is not to match the parameters to some physical quantities, but rather to ensure the desired behavior: force is only active in as small a range as possible, it maintains a reasonable small distance between cells ($\Delta x/2$ in [107]) and it does not lead to numerical instabilities.

To be able to faithfully represent dynamics near contact, the glycocalyx coating of the cells, thermal fluctuations of the membrane and macromolecules (e.g., fibrinogen) in blood plasma would most likely have to be taken into account [70]. Here on the one hand, we face the issue of scarcity of available physiologic data that would enable such modeling and on the other hand the daunting increase in computational complexity in simulations of many cells. For these purposes the simplification using phenomenological repulsive forces seems to be reasonable in both particle-based and mesh-based models.

- **Thermal fluctuations:** Both DPD and LBM-based models are capable of taking into account the thermal fluctuations that influence cell aggregation if the resolution is fine enough. For a healthy cell at rest, instantaneous membrane deflections are around $200nm$ [148] and therefore are not expected to significantly affect the dynamics at the $\sim 10\mu m$ cell scale, except perhaps for particularly close cell-cell interactions mentioned in the previous point.

- **Membrane viscosity:** Including membrane viscosity in the cell models is not straightforward at all. We have seen one approach earlier in this chapter. In particle-based models such as DPD, the viscosity effect is projected onto the connecting vector between two DPD particles as in (3.5). For small velocities, the contribution of the inter-particle relative velocity is negligible, however large values cause numerical instabilities. The remedy for this, presented in [158, Chapter 6], is to consider viscous dissipation force directly proportional to velocity difference:

$$\mathbf{F}_{visc}(A) = -k_{visc}\mathbf{v}_{AB},$$

where k_{visc} is the viscosity coefficient and $\mathbf{v}_{AB}$ is the relative velocity of DPD particles A and B. Analogous force with the opposite sign is assigned to particle B.

Clearly, such an approach is local. It is also force-free, since opposite forces are applied to DPD particles and their resultant is zero. Further, the velocities of the two neighboring mesh points may point in any directions and may have different magnitudes. This means that their difference may be non-zero and that it does not necessarily have to be strictly in-plane or out-of-plane. Consequently, the torque-free condition does not hold in general. Whenever such viscous force is out-of-plane, non-zero torque is applied to the corresponding two particles.

- **Viscosity of inner and outer fluid:** The inner viscosity of the cell is about five times larger than the viscosity of the outer plasma [35]. Together with membrane viscosity, this viscosity difference is the second factor that significantly influences the relaxation of the cell to its resting shape after the cell has experienced deformation. Unlike the IBM and DPD models, the IB-DC model described in this chapter currently does not allow such viscosity difference, since all fluid nodes (including those inside cells) are treated together as one fluid. While it is also possible to technically implement the viscosity difference in the IB-DC model, it has to be done very carefully, because such implementation comes with two major issues.

The first issue is that to locally set the viscosity to a different value in the fluid nodes that are inside blood cells, we need to know that they are inside. This would have to be determined in every time step, since the cells move, while the fluid nodes do not. The fluid nodes that had been inside a cell a moment ago, might no longer be, once the cell has moved. Determining inner points of moving concave objects is possible but it adds to computational complexity.

The second issue is the viscosity drop over the membrane. The discontinuity would lead to dissipation of error and thus inaccuracy of the LB calculations near the cell membrane.

To theoretically compare the membrane elasticity of the spring network, consider the following (detailed calculations provided in the Appendices):

- In all three of these models we have force free and torque-free elastic forces.

- **Stretching:** In the IB-DC model we have a non-linear stretching that corresponds to each mesh edge. In the DPD model, there is either a WLC- or FENE-type spring, both of which are purely attractive. The expansion is taken care of by the DPD area modulus. In the IBM, the surface elastic shear modulus and area dilation modulus are treated together using the Skalak energy model [173].

- **Bending:** The bending forces in the DPD and IBM methods are derived by differentiating the bending energy. In both methods, the bending energy takes the form $E_B = \frac{\kappa_B}{2}(\theta - \theta_0)^2$ that reflects the bending resistance of an elastic sheet defined by Helfrich in [89].

  In the IB-DC method, the forces are defined phenomenologically by (3.8) so that the force-free and torque-free conditions are satisfied. As we have already pointed out at the end of Section 3.4.1, the actual form of the bending forces is identical (up to a multiplicative constant) to that in the DPD and IBM. This can be shown by starting from the bending energy used in DPD and IBM methods $E_B = \frac{\kappa_B}{2}(\theta - \theta_0)^2$ and differentiating it with respect to the positions, as done in Appendix A.2.

- **Local and global area:** Both DPD area forces and IBM global area forces act in the direction of triangle altitudes. They have the largest contribution in the vertex opposite the longest triangle side and the smallest in the vertex that lies opposite the shortest triangle side. For obtuse triangles the expanding area force tends to regularize the triangulation, however, the compression area force will make the triangles even more obtuse, which might lead to numerical problems when dealing with large deformations. The proportional distribution of area forces in the IB-DC model avoids this issue.

  While the directions of local area and global area forces are different in the IB-DC and the other two approaches, the question is whether the energy of these forces is the same when using unit coefficients. The answer to this question is no. More precisely, the energy of area forces in the IB-DC model is exactly twice the energy in the DPD or IBM model. This is derived from the fact that while in the IB-DC model, the relation between area compression modulus and local area coefficient in the absence of stretching forces is $K = k_{al}/2$, for the DPD and for the IBM model it is $K = k_{al}$ [57]. More details are provided in Chapter 4.

- **Volume:** The volume forces are the same in the DPD and IBM models. While the IB-DC forces are out-of-triangle-plane, the DPD/IBM volume forces are not perpendicular and thus also have an in-plane component. Interestingly, after doing the accounting carefully, the resultant applied forces per vertex are the same in all three models, as can be seen in Appendix C.

While two models might theoretically be capable of modeling the same processes, their computational comparison is not straightforward. For example, the elasticity is implemented differently and thus a direct exchange of elastic parameters is not helpful. To make sure that both models work under the same conditions, it is necessary to do the parameter fitting to physical quantities in both models, such as stretching coefficient k_s to the membrane shear modulus μ_0. Other parameters of this kind are for example the bending coefficient k_b, local area coefficient k_{al}, viscosity coefficient k_{visc}, fluid density and viscosity.

Some parameters are artificial but need to be set so that they result in some desired behavior. An example of this kind are the global area coefficient and volume coefficient. They do not correspond to a physical membrane characteristic, but they are here to make sure that the surface and volume of the cell do not vary too much (more than a few percent) since the biological cell has this property. Other parameters of this kind are the local friction coefficient ξ that regulates the cell-fluid interaction and mass (both in our model and in DPD).

When comparing models, dimensionless quantities, especially the Capillary number for blood flows happening at low Reynolds number, are a useful characterisation of flow. These quantities are also suitable identifiers when performing a simulation study with the same model under different conditions.

Dimensionless quantities

The laws of nature cannot depend on a system of units that we choose. Therefore it makes sense to describe the physical system in terms of dimensionless variables. So for a system with physical variables (e.g. density, velocity, viscosity) that can be described using the standard units (e.g. mass, length, time, but in microfluidic models, often length, time and density are used), there are dimensionless quantities that characterise the system. These arise from the fact that there are more physical variables than the fundamental units and the number of these characteristic dimensionless quantities is explicitly expressed by the Buckingham π theorem [18].

For a more detailed and rigorous explanation of non-dimensionalisation, see, e.g. [109]. Here we mention two of the most commonly used dimensionless quantities used to characterise the flow.

This comes with some words of warning though. These definitions are not unique and therefore one should take caution, when comparing them across different models and authors. For example, there is a length variable in the Reynolds number. Some people take this as a particle radius, others the typical length of the system (e.g. width of the channel). Similarly, velocity may be the average/characteristic velocity or the maximum velocity in the system.

Reynolds number

$$Re = \frac{inertial\ force}{viscous\ force} = \frac{\rho \mathbf{v} r}{\mu} = \frac{\rho \dot{\gamma} r^2}{\mu},$$

where ρ is the fluid density, μ is its dynamic viscosity, $\mathbf{v}$ is the characteristic velocity of the fluid, r is particle radius or other typical dimension, and $\dot{\gamma}$ is the shear rate.

Low Reynolds numbers characterise laminar flow and high Re numbers characterise turbulent flow. For $Re \ll 1$, as is the case of blood flow in microcirculation, we not only have laminar flow, but the flow is governed by Stokes law. This means that the viscous (frictional) effects are more dominant than inertial forces.

Capillary number

$$Ca = \frac{viscous\ force}{surface\ tension} = \frac{\mu \mathbf{v}}{\sigma} = \frac{\mu \dot{\gamma} r}{\sigma},$$

where σ is the surface tension.

When modeling elastic objects, it makes sense to replace the surface tension in the denominator with membrane shear elastic modulus μ_0, since we are talking about the capillary number of the cell membrane

$$Ca = \frac{\mu \dot{\gamma} r}{\mu_0}.$$

This means that here the capillary number is a ratio between hydrodynamic stresses due to shearing and stresses due to particle deformation. Note that in dense suspensions, the numerator can be replaced by some quantification of suspension stress, which includes the effect of other cells as well, since it is the combined effect of both the fluid and other cells that this particular cell membrane feels.

At very low capillary number, the surface tension is stronger than the

solver/lab	model(s)	availability
COMSOL multiphysics	continuum CFD, FEM	proprietary
Ansys Fluent	continuum CFD	proprietary
Electric Ant Lab [111]	cell-scale	in-house
YALES2BIO [113, 172]	IBM+continuum CFD	in-house
Kruger Lab [110]	IBM+LBM+FEM	in-house
LAMMPS based [14, 113]	DPD, SDPD	in-house
HemoCell [197]	IBM+LBM+DEM	open-source
OpenRBC [183]	coarse-grained MD	open-source
ESPResSo based	LBM, IBM [73], IB-DC [31]	open-source

TABLE 3.5: Available blood flow solvers. Implementations of models compared in this section are highlighted in **bold**.

---

viscous forces and the object resists being deformed. When a single cell is placed in shear flow, we can observe a transition from tank-treading to tumbling by lowering the capillary number. By increasing it, we see tank-treading with larger elongation of the cell.

For deformable particles in flow, the capillary number is probably more important than the Reynolds number, since we consider all our flow to be laminar at low Re, but it makes sense to distinguish between low ($\sim 10^{-5} - 10^{-2}$) and large (~ 0.1) capillary number.

Once we have both models representing the same setup and corresponding to *bioreality* (more on that in the following chapter), we can think about their comparison regarding computational efficiency (ideally on the same machines) and scalability of the model.

In Table 3.5, we summarise the blood flow solvers available at the time of writing this book. In terms of availability, we divide them into three categories: proprietary, in-house and open-source. Proprietary solvers require purchase of a computational package. Typically they are easier to use, since they include a GUI and integrated visualisation packages. It is more difficult to customize them to perform simulations that are out of their primary scope. In-house solvers include solutions that are either completely custom-made by the research groups or companies or built on existing available packages but not available for public use. Open-source solvers are freely available in the public domain.

Chapter 4

Model vs. bioreality

4.1 Is the model correct?

Everybody who wants to use a model should be concerned whether the model and the results produced with it are *correct*. The meaning of the word *correct* is clear at first sight, but its true meaning can be difficult to characterise. Words like *robust, accurate, reliable, representing the reality* pop up when thinking about it deeper. We can even dig into the literature about the theory of verification and validation of computational models and find out in [167, 170] that, e.g. validation is a *substantiation that a computerised model within its domain of applicability possesses a satisfactory range of accuracy consistent with the intended application of the model.* We try to use simpler words.

For the model to be used, the key element is that the users have confidence in the model. In building such confidence, there are two basic concepts. First, we need to ensure, that

we build the model *right*

and further that

we build the *right* model.

The former concept is supported by the process of model verification and the latter by the process of model validation. Model verification is utilised in the comparison of the conceptual model to the numerical and computer representation that implements that conception. It asks questions like: Did we solve the problem correctly? Is the model implemented correctly from the numerical point of view? What about its implementation in the computer? Are the input parameters and logical structure of the model correctly represented? The typical answers to those questions are: Refine the mesh to see convergence. Verify the numerics. Test the computer code for errors. Model validation is utilised to determine that a model is an accurate representation of the real system. Typical questions that may arise are: Did we solve the right problem? Is the simplification that we made acceptable? Can the simulation results recover the actual real-world behavior? Are the computational results obtained without their direct experimental counterparts sane? The typical responses could be: Such simplification is justified since we are interested in long-term behavior only. Yes, we have fit the experimental data perfectly. Wow, this cannot be true, otherwise Einstein's relativity theory would not be valid, something is not correct. The last response most likely leads back to model verification.

In order to determine the credibility of a computational model, the field of verification and validation has emerged in the engineering and physical sciences communities and it provides formalism, methodologies and best practices for evaluating the reliability of computational models [37].

So to summarise, verification is the process of ensuring that the computational model accurately solves the mathematical model, validation is the process of using data to evaluate the extent that the computational model accurately represents the real-world process, which it attempts to simulate.

4.1.1   Verification

We need to be sure that the code does what it is supposed to do. This is done by confirming that the software correctly implements the required algorithms [37]. For a software, a major aspect of this is confirming that the numerical solution converges to the true solution of the system as discretisation parameters (spatial step and/or time step) are decreased. Ideally, we can check that the convergence is at the rate predicted by the theory.

The main approaches to code verification are to solve problems with known analytic solutions or to compare several independently written codes using a common problem [150]. The former approach allows us to determine exact errors and convergence rates but is usually only possible for simplified (non-physical/non-physiological) problems. The latter approach has the advantage of being feasible on more complex problems but suffers from the lack of a gold-standard solution. The two approaches are complementary and it is important that research fields develop a set of well-defined community-wide benchmark problems, with and without exact solutions, to aid code verification.

Comparisons of codes have been performed, for example, on astronomy codes [68], meteorology codes [6], seismic data processing codes [88] or cardiac electro-physiology codes [141]. While there is a vast literature in several research areas concerning single-cell modeling, we are not aware of any work comparing existing codes or defining benchmarks for whole cell simulation.

Considering the above, we approach verification by suggesting some practices that we think are useful, demonstrated on examples.

Check small pieces of code. This is a general rule, which applies outside cell modeling software as well.

Design simple experiments with outcomes known in advance. If you implement a specific feature, it is good to think of a situation when this feature is pronounced or even isolated and to model this situation. One such example is the viscosity force. This force acts against rapid changes. So make a part of your cell rapidly change and look, whether the generated forces act in the right manner.

Visualise the output. The first sanity check (besides the crashed execution of the simulation code) is to visually inspect the output. Whether it is deformation of a cell, when it should be deformed, rotation of a cell when it should be rotating, or anything else, a visual check gives you a quick answer when something is not right. When implementing the forces, it is useful to see how large these forces are. So for example, one can color the surface of a cell according to the magnitude of individual forces.

Understand there is no such thing as perfect code. It may happen, that even a well-checked source code has a bug. Unfortunately, it is not unreasonable to say that the previous sentence is too optimistic. It should have said that even a well-checked source code has a bug. So if you get strange results, do not assume that all the parts of the code that had been provided by another party (library, physical engine, etc.) are correct and that the bug must be in your code. Sometimes it is not.

Always check using the most simplified computational examples. Every bit of added complexity increases the risk of introducing an error. So try to simplify as much as possible to decrease this risk and to minimise the amount of possible sources of errors. So for example, even if your model incorporates fluid-structure interaction, when checking the implementation of elastic forces, turn the fluid off and check the behavior of the spring network separately.

If you do need to include a more complicated system in your check, do it grad-ually. If you intend to model a system with several different parts, build the system step by step and check each step thoroughly.

Use a priori knowledge. Sometimes, there is prior knowledge of several fea-tures that can be quantified and it can be checked whether the implemented model satisfies it. Good examples are the force-free and torque-free conditions. It is straightforward to implement this check upon the force calculations in the code. Another such example is volume and surface preservation. If a move-ment of a cell involves rotation only, the volume and surface of the cell can be checked. One more such example is symmetry. Once the whole system is symmetrical, it should give symmetrical results too.

4.1.2   Validation

No model is universal. Therefore a model should be developed with *a priori* knowledge of natural phenomena it is intended to mimic. For example, there is no need to use extremely advanced fluid solvers capable of simulating flow with high Reynolds number when we want to simulate flows in microfluidic devices with mostly low to moderate Reynolds numbers. This *a priori* knowledge gives us an estimate of the range of parameters that we want the model to be valid for.

The previous sentence is essentially a concise definition of model *validity*.

To be more specific, let us summarise thoughts from [167]. A model should be developed with a specific application or purpose in mind, and the model validity should be determined by this purpose. The domain of intended appli-cability of the model is defined by numerous sets of experimental conditions. The model may be valid for one set and invalid for another set. To decide whether a model is valid for a set of experimental conditions, the model ac-curacy must be within an acceptable range and this range must be known prior to starting the development of the model or very early in the model development process.

So in an ideal world:

- We know what application we are modeling so that the model is de-veloped for a specific purpose. What is the question we are trying to answer?

- We estimate the range of physical/biological/mechanical parameters so that the domain of the intended applicability of the model is defined.

- We create the model.

- We test whether the model is valid in the specified range so that the model accuracy is within its acceptable range. This is the amount of accuracy required for the intended purpose of the model.

Of course, we do not live in an ideal world and the typical workflow looks more like this:

- The first bullet is easy. We want to simulate, for example, flows of cells in periodic obstacle arrays. Of course, we know what we are modeling.

- The second bullet seems easy, too. We dig into the experimental setups of microarrays and look for fluid flow parameters (volumetric flow rate, fluid velocities, fluid density and viscosity). Then we search for mechanical properties of the cells and we learn about the shear modulus, the area dilatation modulus. And at this point we find out that red blood cells have quite flexible membranes while other cells may have stiff membranes. Since numerics is different for flexible and stiff membranes, we need to decide which kind we are going to model.

Stiff membranes

If a membrane is stiff (but not completely rigid) it features a very strong resistance against deformation. In practical implementation we need to allow for deformability of the membrane and therefore we need to use elastic moduli with high coefficients. This introduces a numerical instability, since forces generated from stiff elastic moduli are much larger than other forces. This means that the time step needs to be smaller to avoid oscillations that can eventually blow up. So even thought one would think that stiff membranes are easier to model, the opposite is true.

- The third bullet requires some work. We build up a model, for example the one from Chapter 3, but in the process of developing the model, we learn that there is maybe an issue with different fluid viscosity inside and outside of the cell membrane. Therefore we go back to bullet two, we search for biological data and learn that sometimes, the viscosity difference is negligible and sometimes it is indeed important. So we adapt the ranges of the parameters, maybe we add another parameter (in this case the viscosity of cell's inner fluid). Then we continue with bullet three. But whoops, we learn that there is a concept of *membrane viscosity*. What is this? Is it important? Under which circumstances? So we go back again to bullet number two and do the research again. And there could be numerous such loopbacks to bullet two. They may always include adding new model details, they might involve adjusting existing features or even removing something that should not have been in the model in the first place.

- If there were any changes in the model in the previous step, the model has to be verified again. And only then are we finally at bullet number four, which is the validation phase. This is the one we specifically talk about in this section. But we have seen that a simple four-bullet list may grow rapidly by several iterations of the second and third (or even the first) bullets.

Things to ponder

If we *only* change the values of the parameters, has the model changed?

What if we use very large values of elastic coefficient and use the model to simulate stiff objects? Is it still the same model?

What if we change the mesh of the cell and use a different triangulation, with the same number of nodes? Has the model changed?

What if we change the mesh of the cell again - this time to a different number of nodes and adjust the dependent values, such as the friction coefficient accordingly? Is this the same model or is it a different one?

What if we implement variable stretching - meaning that for each edge, we can apply a different value of k_s? Has the model changed?

What if we give a different definition of the stretching non-linearity? Has the model changed?

Validation approaches

Biological models often do not have a direct link between the model parameters and the real system parameters. A typical example is the stretching coefficient of the spring network (cell model parameter) and the shear modulus for thin membranes (biological cell parameter). In special cases (e.g. regular triangular meshes), one can derive an explicit expression relating those two parameters. However, in reality, the cell is deformed and even in its relaxed undeformed state, the underlying mesh is not uniform, it has edges with different lengths and at some mesh points it is not regularly triangular. So the explicit expression derived for uniform meshes can, at best, only help us estimate the approximate value of the stretching coefficient.

Therefore, an important part of the validation is the calibration of the model, an iterative process of comparing the model to the real system behavior. The discrepancies between the two and the insights gained from them are used to improve the model. These iterations eventually lead to the values of the model parameters that represent the reality. The process is repeated until the model accuracy is acceptable.

The calibration is mostly done using the available data about the behavior of real systems that are modeled. Besides the calibration, the model must be validated against a different set of data that has *not* been used for calibration. This is because with a sufficiently large parameter space, one can calibrate a model to *any* dataset. The trick is that the calibrated model must comply with other datasets in order to be any good.

There are different techniques for validation of the model [167]. Those that can be used for model calibration are marked with an asterisk.

Animation
The model behavior is displayed graphically as the model moves through time, e.g. the movements of cells passing the obstacles in a microfluidic channel during a simulation run are visualised. The *Animation* approach is very often used as a sanity check whether the model behaves as expected. It is often the first sign of an unusual behavior. It does not prove that the model is right but it can very quickly show that the model is *not right* - by directly showing that something is wrong. Most researchers use animation intuitively and as often as possible.

* Comparison to Other Models
Various results of the simulation model being validated are compared to results of other (valid) models. Where possible, simple cases of a simulation model are compared to known results of analytical models and the simulation model is compared to other simulation models that have been validated.

Comparison to known analytical examples was, for example, used in determining the fluid-structure interaction in Section 3.5. The analytic solution for the movement of a solid ball in a fluid was known and this was used to determine the friction coefficient defining the strength of fluid-structure interaction.

The question of comparing two (or more) computational models is a bit more complicated. Both the observable quantities used for comparison and the scenarios of the computational experiments have to be carefully defined.

Event Validity
Occurrences of specific, not preprogrammed *events* produced by the simulation model are compared to those of the real system to determine if they are similar. For example, the emergence of a cell-free layer near the channel walls is a natural phenomenon and a good cell model should recover this behavior. Besides the cell-free layer, there are more *events* that occur in real-world systems. White blood cell (WBC) margination, shear thinning and rouleaux formation in blood flow are a few examples. Every such *event* has its own characteristics that are observable in laboratory experiments: With the cell-free layer, it is the thickness of the free near-wall layer. With the rouleaux formation, it is the critical shear rate above which the rouleaux vanish. To validate the model, one can simulate the conditions of the experiments and observe whether the *event* occurs and whether the characteristics of the *event* correspond to the observed values from experiments.

Interesting cell behavior in flow

Cell-free layer - A naturally occuring phenomenon, where the elastic red blood cells navigate towards the center of flow, creating a consistent layer free of cells along the boundaries.

Fahraeus-Lindqvist effect - With increasing tube diameter the apparent viscosity of blood flowing inside it is also increasing [67] (with minimum at diameter about $7\mu m$ [59]). This is due to migration of RBCs into the center of the channel and forming the cell-free layer that has lower viscosity and acts as a lubrication between the walls and the bulk of the cells.

Rouleaux formation - Formation of one-dimensional stacks of cells.

Tank-treading - A rolling motion of the membrane about its interior without significant changes of the cell shape.

Shear thinning - Blood viscosity depends on hematocrit, temperature, plasma viscosity, disease state, age of RBCs, etc. At shear rates below $100s^{-1}$, the RBCs affect the blood viscosity [171]. It means that at low shear rates ($\sim 1s^{-1}$), similar cell orientations may favor the formation of rouleaux or 3D clusters of RBCs [156], which both increase the blood viscosity. Above a few $10s^{-1}$, the cells exhibit tank-treading. And at even higher shear rates, the stretching and alignment of the (still tank-treading, but now ellipsoidal) RBCs due to the flow decreases blood viscosity.

Margination - Unlike the RBCs, the white blood cells and platelets are likely to flow closer to the channel walls. This results from their physical size and properties (not as elastic as RBCs) and helps their functions: clotting for platelets and immune response for white blood cells.

---

* Historical Data Validation

There are numerous biological experiments reported in the literature. It is desirable that the model recovers the behavior observed in these experiments. Of course, the parameters of the experiments must lie within the range of validity of the model, otherwise the physics will show up with a vengeance. The foremost advantage of this approach is that no laboratory experiments must be performed, which is clearly very convenient. The risky part is the possible lack of information needed to reproduce the experiment computationally.

Internal Validity

We should make several replications (runs) of a model with different initial conditions to determine the amount of (internal) variability in the model. In real systems, we do not have unique initial conditions: e.g. the same hematocrit in a channel can be achieved by millions of different initial configurations of the cells, or the cells themselves can have different elasticities and we only have data about their averaged values. It is thus crucial that the averaged quantities (such as hematocrit, density of cell, average velocity of the cells in a channel, etc.) remain fairly constant during the simulated process even if the initial configurations are varied (while preserving the initial averaged quantities). Large variability and lack of consistency make the model results questionable. We discuss the methods for random seedings in Section 5.3. Internal validity checks are even more important for stochastic models - those which include probabilistic outcomes even for identical initial conditions. The outcomes should not depend on the stochastic differences in input.

Monitoring Indicators
Values of various indicators of dynamical behavior, e.g. the cell deformation index, are visually displayed as the simulation model runs in time to ensure they behave correctly. One can also monitor performance measures in a similar fashion. Similar to the *Animation* approach, this approach can give a quick information if something goes wrong but it does not give a solid confirmation whether the model is fundamentally sound.

Parameter Variability - Sensitivity Analysis
This technique consists of changing the values of the input and internal parameters of a model to determine the effect of such change upon the model behavior and output. The same outcomes should be observed in the model as in the real system. Those parameters that are sensitive, i.e. cause significant changes in the model behavior or output, should be made sufficiently accurate prior to using the model. (This may require further iterations of the model development.) For example, in stretching experiments, the bending coefficient influences the final stretched length of a cell much less than the stretching and local area coefficients. An example of sensitivity analysis can be found in Section 3.5.5, where we determine the most influential model parameters for the calibration of fluid-structure interaction.

Predictive Validation
The model is used to predict (forecast) the system behavior and then the actual system behavior is compared to the prediction. The system data may come from experiments reported in the literature or by conducting new laboratory experiments. *Predictive Validation* is one of the strongest approaches in building the confidence in a model. If a model can effectively predict the behavior, against which it has not been tested or calibrated, this tells us that the model really captures the modeled system.

4.2   What does the theory of membrane mechanics tell us?

Before we dive into the concepts of membrane mechanics and fluid flow, we need to discuss some theoretical aspects. The first step in model validation is linking the model parameters to real system parameters. The physical parameters of the fluid enter the lattice-Boltzmann method directly. Parameters such as fluid density and fluid viscosity are available in the literature for any physical fluid used in the experiments, and we can use these values in the model (after proper unit scaling). More details are available in Appendix F.

Elastic parameters however are more complicated. In Chapter 3 we have gradually built a mesh-based model with one viscous and five elastic parameters, namely the stretching, bending, local and global area, volume and viscosity coefficients. Our real system, on the other hand, is a cell and we adopted the notion that this cell is represented only by its membrane, which separates its inner cytoplasm from the surrounding fluid. Therefore, the whole (visco-) elasticity is represented by the (visco-) elasticity of the membrane.

In order to link the model parameters to the real system parameters, we first need to understand our real system and its mechanics.

4.2.1   Mechanics of the continuum model for a membrane

The membrane of a cell (e.g. of a red blood cell) consists of several components. The interplay among them results in elastic behavior of the membrane, which can be modeled by continuum mechanics, where the membrane is treated as an isotropic thin sheet. Such a continuum model has several elastic parameters, and those parameters are often estimated from dedicated biological experiments.

There is however a difference in the nature of the in-plane and out-of-plane moduli. We discuss each of them individually. Before we do that, let us briefly agree on some notions in membrane mechanics.

Basic notions

Consider a two-dimensional object under the influence of some external forces, depicted in Figure 4.1. Make a cross section by an arbitrary line and look at the force **F** that acts upon the cross section. This force can be split into a normal direction that is perpendicular to the cross-secting line, magnitude of the normal component denoted by F_n, and tangential direction along the cross section, magnitude of the tangential component denoted by F_t. Now we can distinguish between two stresses that act upon the cross section: the *normal stress* defined as F_n/L and tangential stress, or *shear stress*, defined as F_t/L.

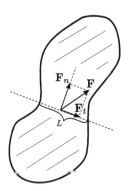

FIGURE 4.1: Normal and tangential forces acting upon a body cross-section in 2D.

Now we can consider a deformation caused by a force. To keep it simple, we assume linear elastic deformation. In Figure 4.2, we can see some examples of such deformation. In (a), we see pure shear deformation, in (b) we see isotropic area expansion in all directions. In the case of pure shear, the normal stress along the y-direction (in such rectangular setting) is denoted by $\sigma_{yy} = 0$. Analogously, the normal stress in the x-direction is denoted by $\sigma_{xx} = 0$. The shear stress in y-direction is denoted by τ_{xy} and is given by $\tau_{xy} = F/L_y$. To quantify how much the object was deformed by such shearing, *strain* is defined as relative change of lengths. Here, $\Delta_x L_y$ defines the size of deformation. The subscript x next to Δ refers to the fact that the change is in the x-direction and the subscript y next to L tells us that this deformation is relative to the size of the object in the y-direction. In this case, the *shear strain* is defined as ratio $\epsilon_{xy} = \Delta_x L_y / L_y$. Analogous shear strain $\epsilon_{yx} = \Delta_y L_x / L_x$ is defined when a force in y-direction acts upon the side parallel to y-direction.

In the case of isotropic area expansion in Figure 4.2 (b), the forces act in directions normal to the four sides of a rectangle. They cause the change $\Delta_x L_x$ in x-direction and $\Delta_y L_y$ in y-direction. The *normal strain* is defined as $\epsilon_{xx} = \Delta_x L_x / L_x$ and $\epsilon_{yy} = \Delta_y L_y / L_y$. When an area compressibility is in question, the following relative *area compression* (or *area expansion*) is defined Δ_A / A, where Δ_A is the difference between the stretched and the relaxed surface area of the membrane. In Figure 4.2 (b), the relation

$$\Delta_A = (L_x + \Delta_x L_x)(L_y + \Delta_y L_y) - L_x L_y$$

holds.

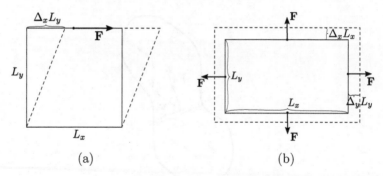

FIGURE 4.2: (a) Shear deformation and (b) isotropic expansion of a 2D rectangular sheet.

General in-plane elastic moduli

Elastic objects undergoing deformations react by internal stresses. Their resistance to the deformation is characterised by different *elastic moduli*. The deformation is often caused by complex forces and to simplify the quantification of elastic resistance, those complex forces are split into simple cases. Assuming the linearity of such resistance - with small deformations, this is a reasonable assumption - the approach to quantify such resistance follows these steps:

1. Define a simple deformation, giving the strain

2. Deform the material

3. Measure the forces caused by the material trying to get back to its original shape

4. Compute the resulting stress

5. Define the deformation modulus corresponding to the particular simple deformation by the formula

$$stress = modulus \cdot strain$$

Unlike their 3D counterparts, the in-plane deformations of 2D membranes involve only two fundamental modes mentioned above: compression (or equivalently expansion) and shear.

In the following, we discuss these two modes.

Shear mode

Following the steps from the previous section, we first choose pure shear as a deformation. Then according to the second step, we deform the rectangular sheet of material as depicted in Figure 4.2 (a). This introduces strain $\epsilon_{xy} = \Delta_x L_y / L_y$. Thirdly, the deformation causes the force F acting to restore the material to its original shape. As the fourth step, we have the resulting shear stress given by $\tau_{xy} = F/L_x$. Finally, the shear modulus denoted by μ_0 is defined by

$$\tau_{xy} = \mu_0 \epsilon_{xy}, \quad \mu_0 = \frac{F L_y}{\Delta_x L_y L_x}.$$

The rectangular sheet however only seldom deforms to a rectangle. Therefore we adopt the infinitesimal computation of μ_0 by differentiating the first relation above with respect to ϵ_{xy}, leading to

$$\mu_0 = \frac{d\tau_{xy}}{d\epsilon_{xy}}\bigg|_{\epsilon_{xy}=0}. \tag{4.1}$$

Such expression has been used numerous times, e.g. in [40, 56].

Area compression/expansion mode

In order to derive the definition of the area expansion modulus, we modify the second step. First we again choose an isotropic extension of a square as a simple deformation. Then in the second step, we deform the square. We are interested in area expansion so for the computation of strain, we do not consider the relative change in length but rather the relative change in the area of the square $\epsilon = \Delta A / A_0 = (A - A_0)/A_0$, where A_0 is the relaxed area of the square and A is the area of the stretched square. In step 3, we measure the restoring forces F. Forces are normal to all four sides of the square and therefore the stresses in step 4 are normal stresses $\sigma_{xx} = \sigma_{yy} = F/L$. Total normal stress is their average $P = (\sigma_{xx} + \sigma_{yy})/2$. When using Figure 4.2 (b), we have $L_x = L_y = L$.

Finally, the deformation modulus K called *area compression* or *area expansion* modulus is then defined by

$$P = \frac{1}{2}(\sigma_{xx} + \sigma_{yy}) = K \frac{A - A_0}{A_0}.$$

Again, the square is deformed to a square only in the infinitesimal limit, so we compute K by differentiating the previous relation with respect to A:

$$K = A_0 \frac{dP}{dA}\bigg|_{A=A_0}, \tag{4.2}$$

as used also in [40, 56].

Why are the two relations different?
We have obtained two relations, one for shear modulus (4.1) and one for area compression modulus (4.2), and they differ in multiplication by A_0 in the latter one. This difference came from the fact that the relation for area compression was differentiated with respect to the area and not with

respect to the strain. Otherwise, the relation for area compression would be

$$K = \frac{dP}{d\epsilon}\bigg|_{\epsilon=0},$$

and would correspond to the relation with shear modulus. We chose this form to conform to the common usage in the literature.

Young's modulus and Poisson's ratio
In the theory of elastic deformation, Young's modulus defines a measure of a material stiffness. To be more precise, it is the ratio of stress along an axis to the strain along that axis. Young's modulus is often denoted by Y.

When 2D sheets are stretched, they prolong in axial direction and contract in the transversal direction. The ratio of relative contraction to relative prolongation is called *Poisson's ratio* and is often denoted by ν.

Both Young's modulus and Poisson's ratio are connected to the shear modulus and area compressibility of 2D sheets by the following relations [15]:

$$Y = \frac{4K/\mu_0}{K + \mu_0}, \qquad \nu = \frac{K - \mu_0}{K + \mu_0}.$$

Out-of-plane bending mode

In the previous text, we have discussed the in-plane deformations. However, the lipid bilayer of red blood cell membranes also leads to the membrane resistance to bending [135]. The bilayer consists of two neighboring sheets of elongated lipid molecules, whose axes are oriented perpendicularly to the membrane surface. Their hydrophilic heads point outwards, towards the aqueous surrounding, while the hydrophobic tails are oriented towards the membrane interior. Different forms of the bending energy have been proposed in the past, all depending on the square of the mean curvature, [52, 89] and other references in [82]. One of the most popular models dates back to Helfrich, where the total bending energy stored in the infinitesimally thin interface is given by

$$E_b = \frac{k_c}{2} \int (C_1 + C_2 - 2C_0)^2 dA. \tag{4.3}$$

Here, C_1 and C_2 are the local principal curvatures, C_0 is the spontaneous curvature and k_C is the bending rigidity. For spherical membranes with radius R, local curvatures are given by $C_1 = C_2 = 1/R$.

In-plane viscous mode

Viscous forces are difficult to measure, since viscosity is *visible* only through its damping effect on other phenomena. For example, if pure stretching is involved, after release a viscoelastic material would contract with a specific speed. The larger the viscosity, the slower is this speed. Therefore, the viscosity is often determined from experiments indirectly through measuring the amount of the other phenomena that have decreased within a given time period.

In our case, consider a spring with the shear modulus μ_0. With generated strain ϵ, the resulting stress τ would be given by

$$\tau = \mu_0 \epsilon.$$

Viscosity takes into account the dynamics of the deformation. Therefore, the general formula for the viscosity modulus must be adapted by using the time derivative

$$stress = modulus \cdot \frac{d(strain)}{dt}.$$

So in the case of viscous force, when a small deformation from the relaxed state causes strain ϵ, we can release the spring and measure time Δt until the spring gets back to the relaxed state. Using the previous relation, the stress is then given by

$$\tau = \eta_m \frac{\epsilon}{\Delta t},$$

where η_m denotes the *viscosity modulus*. Combining the two equations for stress, we come to

$$\eta_m = \mu_0 \Delta t.$$

This relation has been used to estimate membrane viscosity indirectly from measurements of cell relaxation time after stretching [93, 122].

Transition from continuum formulation to discrete formulation
Consider the following analogy: derivative and its approximation. For a smooth function f one can compute its derivative at a given point x_0 by computing the limit

$$f'(x_0) = \lim_{h \to 0} \frac{f(x_0 + h) - f(x_0)}{h}.$$

Using equidistant discretisation by points $x_1, x_2, \ldots, x_i, x_{i+1}, \ldots$ with discretisation step h, one can approximate the derivative by the following expression:

$$f'(x_i) \approx \frac{f(x_{i+1}) - f(x_i)}{h}.$$

In the case of a 1D derivative, it was fairly easy to approximate the continuous quantity (derivative) by its discrete counterpart for a given spatial discretisation.

In our 2D case, we also have a continuous quantity and a spatial discretisation:

- *Pressure*

We have relations (4.1) and (4.2) that are continuous expressions involving *stress*; it is shear stress in (4.1) and sum of normal stresses in (4.2). In both cases, the shear stress and normal stresses represent pressure.

- *Spring network*
  Our discretisation of space is the triangular network of springs with given elastic moduli.

So a natural step forward is to derive the discrete counterparts of shear stress and normal stresses so that we can relate them. After general considerations about pressure in a spring network system, we derive microscopic pressure around one point in such network because the relations (4.1) and (4.2) are pointwise.

4.2.2   Pressure in the spring network system

A spring network can be considered as a system of mass points occupying volume V with position vectors $\mathbf{r}_i$, point masses m_i and velocities $\mathbf{v}_i$. There are forces acting between these points, which are either two-body forces (acting between two points, depending on their relative position), three-body forces (acting among three points, depending on the relative positions of the three points), or possibly four- or more-body forces. For each point, the sum of all forces acting on this point is denoted by $\mathbf{F}_i$.

Virial theorem
The virial theorem (4.4) provides a general way to relate the total kinetic and potential energy of a stable system with many particles bound by potential forces.

This system has its kinetic and potential energy. Kinetic energy comes from the movement of the mass and is computed simply by summing up the $m_i(\mathbf{v}_i, \mathbf{v}_i)/2$ terms. The potential energy is more sophisticated. The virial theorem however simplifies the computation. The relation (1) in [42] states that microscopic pressure is given by

$$P = \frac{1}{3V}\left(\sum_i m_i(\mathbf{v}_i, \mathbf{v}_i) + \sum_i (\mathbf{r}_i, \mathbf{F}_i)\right) \tag{4.4}$$

The last term is called the *virial* of the system and we denote it by $\mathcal{W}$. If the system is not moving and only feels some tension from external forces, the kinetic part of the previous equation vanishes and we have the following relation for the pressure:

$$P = \frac{1}{3V}\sum_i (\mathbf{r}_i, \mathbf{F}_i),$$

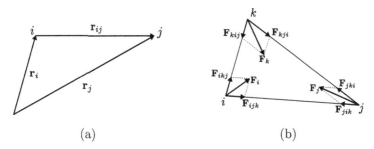

(a)   (b)

FIGURE 4.3: (a) Position vectors vs. relative vectors. (b) Three-body forces decomposed onto the edges.

where V is the volume of the examined system.

Our spring network system is a closed 2D surface in three dimensions that represents the cell membrane, therefore we start the discussion with a planar 2D system occupying area A, where the pressure is

$$P = \frac{1}{2A} \sum_i (\mathbf{r}_i, \mathbf{F}_i). \tag{4.5}$$

Let us compute virial for the case of two-body forces only. Assume that the mutual forces between two points i, j are always attractive or repulsive, which means that they act along the vector between points i, j.

$$W = \sum_i (\mathbf{r}_i, \mathbf{F}_i) = \sum_i (\mathbf{r}_i, \sum_{j \neq i} \mathbf{F}_{ij}) = \sum_i \sum_{j > i} ((\mathbf{r}_i, \mathbf{F}_{ij}) + (\mathbf{r}_j, \mathbf{F}_{ji})),$$

where $\mathbf{F}_{ij}$ denotes the force acting on point i under the influence of point j. Two-body forces are symmetrical so we have $\mathbf{F}_{ij} = -\mathbf{F}_{ji}$ and thus we end up with

$$W = \sum_i \sum_{j > i} ((\mathbf{r}_i - \mathbf{r}_j), \mathbf{F}_{ij}) = \sum_i \sum_{j > i} (\mathbf{r}_{ij}, \mathbf{F}_{ij}), \tag{4.6}$$

where we have replaced position vectors $\mathbf{r}_i$ and $\mathbf{r}_j$ by relative vector $\mathbf{r}_{ij} = \mathbf{r}_i - \mathbf{r}_j$ as depicted in Figure 4.3 (a).

In the three-body case, we assume that the forces $\mathbf{F}_i, \mathbf{F}_j, \mathbf{F}_k$ resulting from the mutual interaction of points i, j, k can be split into six forces acting along the edges of triangle ijk, see Figure 4.3 (b). Given three points i, j, k, let us denote $\mathbf{F}_{ijk}$ the force acting on point i along the vector ij, with obvious analogy for $\mathbf{F}_{ikj}, \mathbf{F}_{jik}$, etc.

In the following we assume that the magnitudes of forces acting along the same triangle edge are the same, so $\mathbf{F}_{ijk} = -\mathbf{F}_{jik}$. We can now compute the

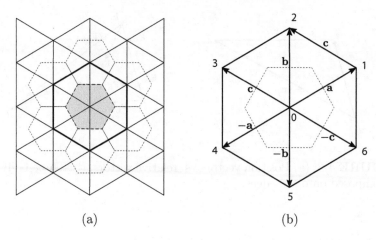

FIGURE 4.4: (a) Uniform triangular mesh depicted with full lines with reference areas corresponding to the vertices and indicated by dashed lines. (b) Six equilateral triangles around one point in triangular mesh.

virial:

$$\mathcal{W} = \sum_i (\mathbf{r}_i, \mathbf{F}_i) = \sum_i (\mathbf{r}_i, \sum_{j \neq i} \sum_{k \neq i, k \neq j} \mathbf{F}_{ijk})$$

$$= \sum_i \sum_{j>i} \sum_{k \neq i, k \neq j} ((\mathbf{r}_i, \mathbf{F}_{ijk}) + (\mathbf{r}_j, \mathbf{F}_{jik})).$$

Now using $\mathbf{F}_{ijk} = -\mathbf{F}_{jik}$ we end up with

$$\mathcal{W} = \sum_i \sum_{j>i} \sum_{k \neq i, k \neq j} ((\mathbf{r}_i - \mathbf{r}_j), \mathbf{F}_{ijk}) = \sum_i \sum_{j>i} (\mathbf{r}_{ij}, \sum_{k \neq i, k \neq j} \mathbf{F}_{ijk}). \qquad (4.7)$$

Note that the sum $\sum_{k \neq i, k \neq j} \mathbf{F}_{ijk}$ in the last expression only has two terms: one for some k_1 and another for some k_2, because in 2D there are exactly two triangles adjacent to one edge. If we were discretising 3D space, the formula would still be valid, but there would be more triangles adjacent to this edge.

4.2.3 Microscopic pressure around one point

In the grey box at the end of Section 4.2.1, we have explained why we want to evaluate the discrete microscopic pressure around one point in a spring network. Let us thus compute the virial around one such point in a uniform triangular network. Figure 4.4 (a) depicts part of such a network with reference areas (represented by dashed lines) that are assigned to the corresponding mesh points. Detail of the network with triangles adjacent to one mesh point is shown in Figure 4.4 (b). Using the notation from the figure, we compute the stress around the central point 0 from (4.6) as

$$P_0 = \frac{1}{2A}[(\mathbf{a}, \mathbf{F}_{01}) + (\mathbf{b}, \mathbf{F}_{02}) + (\mathbf{c}, \mathbf{F}_{03}) + (-\mathbf{a}, \mathbf{F}_{04}) + (-\mathbf{b}, \mathbf{F}_{05}) + (-\mathbf{c}, \mathbf{F}_{06})],$$

where $A = 2S_\triangle$. Since $\mathbf{F}_{01} = -\mathbf{F}_{04} =: \mathbf{F}_a$, and similarly for other pairs of vectors, we get

$$P_0 = \frac{1}{2S_\triangle}\left[(\mathbf{a}, \mathbf{F}_a) + (\mathbf{b}, \mathbf{F}_b) + (\mathbf{c}, \mathbf{F}_c)\right].$$

Following the reasoning in derivation of [56, expression (8)] or [40, expression (3.9)], we deduce the individual components of stress tensor τ_{xy} as

$$\tau_{xy} = \frac{1}{2S_\triangle}\left[\frac{F_a}{a}a_x a_y + \frac{F_b}{b}b_x b_y + \frac{F_c}{c}c_x c_y\right], \tag{4.8}$$

where $a = |\mathbf{a}|, \mathbf{a} = [a_x, a_y], F_a = |\mathbf{F}_a|$ and similarly for other vectors.

In the case of three-body forces we can compute stress around point 0 from (4.7) as

$$\begin{aligned}
P_0 &= \frac{1}{2A}\Big[(\mathbf{a}, \mathbf{F}_{012} + \mathbf{F}_{016}) + (\mathbf{b}, \mathbf{F}_{023} + \mathbf{F}_{021}) + (\mathbf{c}, \mathbf{F}_{034} + \mathbf{F}_{032}) \\
&\quad + (-\mathbf{a}, \mathbf{F}_{045} + \mathbf{F}_{043}) + (-\mathbf{b}, \mathbf{F}_{056} + \mathbf{F}_{054}) + (-\mathbf{c}, \mathbf{F}_{061} + \mathbf{F}_{065})\Big].
\end{aligned}$$

Again, we have the symmetry $\mathbf{F}_{012} = -\mathbf{F}_{045}, \mathbf{F}_{016} = -\mathbf{F}_{043}$, and analogous expressions with shifted indices, so we get

$$P_0 = \frac{1}{2S_\triangle}\Big[(\mathbf{a}, \mathbf{F}_{012} + \mathbf{F}_{016}) + (\mathbf{b}, \mathbf{F}_{023} + \mathbf{F}_{021}) + (\mathbf{c}, \mathbf{F}_{034} + \mathbf{F}_{032})\Big]$$

and

$$\tau_{xy} = \frac{1}{2S_\triangle}\left[\frac{F_{012} + F_{016}}{a}a_x a_y + \frac{F_{023} + F_{021}}{b}b_x b_y + \frac{F_{034} + F_{032}}{c}c_x c_y\right]. \tag{4.9}$$

4.2.4 Relation between model and system parameters

In Section 4.2.1, we have discussed continuum mechanics of a membrane. We know what data we can expect from experimental biologists: shear modulus, area compression/expansion modulus and bending modulus. We model the membrane using a spring network and we need to find out what is the shear, area compression and bending moduli of such a membrane.

In Chapter 3, we have introduced five elastic moduli although we do not know, whether their coefficients $k_s, k_b, k_{al}, k_{ag}, k_v$ correspond to any of μ_0, K, k_c, yet. In our model, we have a clear distinction between local forces and global forces. In biological reality, this distinction is somewhat blurred.

There are numerous experimental methods for identification of area expansion modulus of a membrane, such as micropipette aspiration [129] or optical tweezer stretching [114]. During these experiments, the whole cell is involved and thus global effects do play a role even in determination of local area expansion characteristics of the membrane. Therefore, the linking of model parameters to experimental data must be done with great care.

To determine the relation between continuum parameters and spring network parameters we perform similar steps on the spring network as we have before on the continuum membrane. This time though, we distinguish between the in-plane and out-of-plane scenarios. For the in-plane case:

- We define and apply a simple deformation.

- Deformation induces forces in the system that are functions of k_s, k_{al}, k_{ag}.

- Induced forces quantify the stress in the network as a function of k_s, k_{al}, k_{ag}.

- Knowing the relations between stress and continuum parameters (4.1) and (4.2), we eventually obtain relations between continuum parameters and spring network parameters.

The out-of-plane case includes the analysis of bending modulus and will be discussed later in this chapter.

Before taking any further steps, we emphasise that we assume a regular triangular network as depicted in Figure 4.5. Why are we making such a strong assumption of regularity? The reason is that the subsequent analytical considerations resulting in linking of continuum and spring network parameters may be done only for uniform meshes.

The assumption is not unreasonable though, since even if in practice we use non-uniform meshes resulting from triangulation of real curved surfaces (such as the membrane of a red blood cell), we try to have them as regular as possible. Doing this, we hope to have at least an approximation of relations between continuum and network parameters. And we do not use the derived relations as something fixed. We rather use them as a good starting point for later improvements of model parameters, e.g. by using different validation approaches. We elaborate on this more later.

In-plane shear mode

Since the 2D continuum model for the membrane has only two deformation modes and our spring network model has to reproduce both, we copy the same approach. We start with the simplest deformation, the shear modulus.

In the following text, we show some computations, without writing out all the steps and manual derivations. These are provided in Appendix D.

Following the steps of the previous bullet list, we first use a simple deformation: in this case shear deformation induced by an incremental engineering

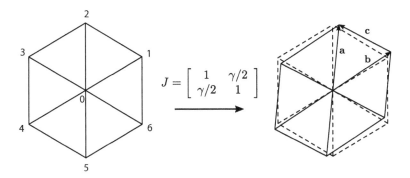

FIGURE 4.5: Undeformed elements of a regular triangular mesh are deformed under the shear deformation given by J. The deformation depicted on the right was obtained with $\gamma = 0.2$.

shear strain γ on the triangular network. This means that the transformation matrix is

$$J = \begin{bmatrix} 1 & \gamma/2 \\ \gamma/2 & 1 \end{bmatrix}$$

and the deformation is given simply by $\mathbf{r} = \mathbf{r}_0 J$. Under this deformation, the vectors $\mathbf{a}_0 = l_0[\frac{\sqrt{3}}{2}, \frac{1}{2}]$, $\mathbf{b}_0 = l_0[0, 1]$, where l_0 is the relaxed length of the vectors, change into vectors $\mathbf{a} = l_0[\frac{\sqrt{3}}{2} + \frac{\gamma}{4}, \frac{1}{2} + \frac{\sqrt{3}\gamma}{4}]$, $\mathbf{b} = l_0[\frac{\gamma}{2}, 1]$ and the other network points change correspondingly. The network is deformed, the lengths of the edges between the mesh points change too and thus there are forces generated in the network. The magnitudes of forces can be calculated as functions of k_s and γ:

$$
\begin{aligned}
F_a &= k_s(a - a_0) = k_s l_0 \gamma \frac{\sqrt{3}}{4} + o(\gamma^2), \\
F_b &= k_s(b - b_0) = o(\gamma^2), \\
F_c &= k_s(c - c_0) = -k_s l_0 \gamma \frac{\sqrt{3}}{4} + o(\gamma^2).
\end{aligned}
$$

Remember, the detailed computations can be found in Appendix D.

Exclusion of other local forces

In these calculations, we ignore the bending forces, which is natural, since there is no out-of-plane deformation. We also ignore the local area forces. The reason for this will be explained later, but a brief explanation is that local area forces will not have any influence on shear resistance of spring network.

Such forces induce stress in the network. Since they are coming only from the stretching of the network, these forces are thus two-body interactions between the nodes of triangular lattice. Denoting them $\mathbf{F}_a, \mathbf{F}_b, \mathbf{F}_c$ they act between the origin and endpoints of vectors $\mathbf{a}, \mathbf{b}, \mathbf{c}$, respectively. From the theory of microscopic pressure around one point in a network presented in Section 4.2.3, we have expression (4.8) for τ_{xy} around a mesh point located at origin

$$\tau_{xy} = \frac{1}{2A} \left[\frac{F_a}{a} a_x a_y + \frac{F_b}{b} b_x b_y + \frac{F_c}{c} c_x c_y \right]$$

Plugging in the expressions for coordinates of $\mathbf{a}, \mathbf{b}, \mathbf{c}$ and for the magnitudes F_a, F_b, F_c we end up with the expression for τ_{xy} as a function of k_s and γ.

Since the shear stress in membranes is defined from (4.1) as

$$\mu_0 = \left. \frac{d\tau_{xy}}{d\gamma} \right|_{\gamma=0},$$

our next step is to compute the derivative. Using (for example) the automatic differentiation tool we end up with the final expression

$$\mu_0 = \left. \frac{d\tau_{xy}}{d\gamma} \right|_{\gamma=0} = k_s \frac{\sqrt{3}}{4}. \tag{4.10}$$

This same relation has been derived in other works, e.g. [15, (5.24)].

There is a reasonably good consensus in the literature about the value of μ_0. The values of shear modulus obtained using the micropipette aspiration technique were $\mu_0 = 7.5 \pm 1.5 \mu N/m$ in [92] and $\mu_0 = 7.98 \mu N/m$ in [40]. Slightly lower values were obtained by optical tweezers experiments in [91], where $\mu_0 = 2.5 \pm 0.4 \mu N/m$. The review paper [186] combines data from several approaches and gives the range $\mu_0 = 5.5 \pm 3.3 \mu N/m$.

Before using the formula (4.10) to calculate the value of k_s in the model, remember that there were three assumptions that we have relied on in the calculation: it holds for linear stretching, for planar mesh and for perfectly regular triangulation - equilateral triangles.

Why can we exclude the area forces from the calculation of k_s?
We need to pay the debt here. In the previous box we have said it is not necessary to consider local area forces when incremental engineering shear strain is applied to a spring network. Why is that?

Local area forces act as soon as the surface of a triangle changes from its relaxed value. Well, in Appendix D we have computed the area of deformed triangles to be $A = A_0 + o(\gamma^2)$. So the area does change. Luckily, in the expression (4.10), after differentiation with respect to γ the quadratic contribution from local area forces would remain linearly dependent of γ and thus when evaluating the derivative at $\gamma = 0$, the contribution vanishes.

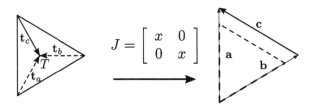

FIGURE 4.6: Undeformed triangular element of a regular triangular mesh is deformed under isotropic expansion given by J. The deformation depicted on the right was obtained with $x = 1.2$.

In-plane area compression/expansion mode

To analyse the second deformation mode acting in 2D, we apply isotropic network expansion given by

$$J = \begin{bmatrix} x & 0 \\ 0 & x \end{bmatrix}.$$

The deformation is defined by parametrisation with parameter $x \geq 0$, with $x = 1$ corresponding to the relaxed state. In Figure 4.6 we see one triangle of the regular triangular network deformed under such expansion.

Again, we are going to follow the steps from the previous bullet list. Applying isotropic expansion for $x > 1$, we get a deformed network. The new coordinates of the mesh points are

$$\mathbf{a} = \left[\frac{\sqrt{3}}{2} x l_0, \frac{1}{2} x l_0 \right], \quad \mathbf{b} = [0, x l_0].$$

Other lengths and areas can be evaluated too, but we again relegate the details to Appendix D for brevity.

In the case of isotropic expansion, the lengths of the edges change as well as the area of triangle surface. Therefore, the forces generated by this deformation come from three network moduli: stretching, local area and global area. The stretching of the edges induces two-body forces modeled by linear springs with stiffness k_s and relaxed length l_0, so we have the following magnitudes of forces:

$$F_a = F_b = F_c = k_s(x - 1)l_0.$$

The local area expansion defines forces given by (3.4). These forces however are not two-body forces. Local area force is bound to a triangle and thus it is a three-body force. The same holds for global area forces. Together with the previous relation for F_a, F_b, F_c we obtain an expression for two-body and three-body forces as a function of k_s, k_{al}, k_{ag} and x.

These forces can be plugged into computation of the normal stresses in the network. Consequently, the relations (4.8) and (4.9) apply and after (very) tedious computations we can arrive at the following result for diagonal pressure:

$$P = \frac{1}{2}(\sigma_{xx} + \sigma_{yy}) = k_s\sqrt{3}\frac{x-1}{x} + \frac{k_{al}}{2}\frac{x^2-1}{x^2} + \frac{k_{ag}}{2}(x^2-1).$$

Details of the derivations are present in Appendix D. So we have just quantified the stress in the network as function of k_s, k_{al}, k_{ag} and x.

We know how the pressure is related to the area compression modulus (in the continuum model) by (4.2). Here, the dependence is expressed with variable A, while in the above expression for P we have dependence on x. Using the chain rule and the fact that $A = cl_0^2 x^2$ we can get that

$$A_0\frac{dP}{dA} = A_0\frac{dP}{dx}\frac{dx}{dA} = A_0\frac{dP}{dx}\frac{1}{2cxl_0^2} = A_0\frac{dP}{dx}\frac{x}{2A_0} = \frac{dP}{dx}\frac{x}{2}.$$

We differentiate P with respect to x and we finally obtain

$$K = k_s\frac{\sqrt{3}}{2} + \frac{k_{al}}{2} + \frac{k_{ag}}{2}. \tag{4.11}$$

Does global area really contribute to area expansion modulus?
Theoretical calculus from Appendix D, which gives the relation (4.11) assumes regular expansions of the mesh under consideration. This means that all triangles in the mesh are expanded equally. In such a case, the derived relation (4.11) holds. But how do we get such mesh expansion in reality? The closest we can get is the case of a nearly regular mesh of an isotropically expanded sphere. Therefore, when using the relation (4.11), the physiological value of K needs to be obtained from the experiment, in which the whole cell was isotropically expanded.

However, the experiments described later are not of such a nature. Micropipette aspiration, as well as dynamic membrane fluctuations, do not achieve isotropic cell expansion. Therefore the global area forces are only partially present in such experiments, and for linking of the expansion modulus and spring network parameters we use only local forces, namely stretching and local area forces. The corresponding relation thus simplifies to

$$K = k_s\frac{\sqrt{3}}{2} + \frac{k_{al}}{2}. \tag{4.12}$$

To account for global area forces, in practice we maintain the global surface area fluctuations below 1%.

When one wants to find the biological values of area compression modulus K, the situation is more complicated than in case of the shear modulus. Micropipette aspiration measurements give values $K = 450mN/m$ [193] or $K = 353 \pm 121mN/m$ [129], which are also reflected in the range

$K = 399 \pm 110 mN/m$ given in the review paper [186]. Note that these numbers are several orders of magnitude larger than the values of μ_0.

Other measurements have been done using dynamic membrane fluctuations [149] and these give range $K = 0.01 - 0.1 mN/m$. In the paper, they explain the inconsistency by saying that there is strong strain stiffening in the membrane as the membrane fluctuations are removed by an applied tension in the micropipette aspiration technique.

Yet another approach is theoretical and used in [40, 56], where they demonstrate that K should be approximately two times larger than μ_0. This has been experimentally verified in [114], where they have measured the area compression modulus of the spectrin skeleton of the membrane. Quantitatively, this would correspond to the dynamic membrane fluctuations results. The micropipette aspiration technique apparently also takes into account the properties of the lipid bilayer and in its scope is a much more global, not local measurement.

Therefore for our model, we can take the approach of setting $k_{al} = 2k_s$ and setting k_{ag} to correspond to $K = 0.4N/m$. Note, that such a value of k_{ag} might be too large from a numerical perspective (too stiff problem that would require too small time step) and therefore for practical purposes it makes sense to make k_{ag} just large enough that the total surface of the simulated cell does not change above a predefined threshold, e.g. 1% deviation from a relaxed state.

Why did we get a different $K - k_{al}$ relation than in the DPD and IBM models?

In Section 3.7.2 we highlight the similarities and differences of our IB-DC model and other two models: DPD and IBM. One of the differences is that the relation between K and k_{al}, k_{ag} is different in the IB-DC model compared to DPD and IBM. Both of these have the same relation:

$$K = k_d + k_a,$$

under assumption of zero stretching forces, where k_d is the DPD local area coefficient and k_a is the global area coefficient. An interesting point is that compared to (4.11), this relation is missing a division by two.

There is however a good explanation for this. Consider local area forces only. If one explicitly computes DPD local area forces in an expanded equilateral triangle (for detailed computations see Appendix D.3), the result is

$$|\mathbf{F}_{DPD}| = k_d \frac{(x^2 - 1)}{2} x l_0,$$

while in the IB-DC case we have

$$|\mathbf{F}_{IB-DC}| = k_{al} \frac{(x^2 - 1)}{4x} l_0.$$

There are two differences between expressions for $\mathbf{F}_{DPD}$ and $\mathbf{F}_{IB-DC}$: The first one is that the term x appears once in the numerator and once in the denominator. Now when we are considering small changes, that is $x \approx 1$, this difference does not play a big role and, in consecutive differentiations evaluated at $x = 1$, this difference does not play any role at all.

The second difference is the division by two in one case and by four in the other. This basically means that IB-DC local area forces are one half of the DPD forces. So to have the same impact on the spring network, the IB-DC model needs to use twice as high a value of the local area modulus than DPD. In symbols we thus have

$$k_{al} = 2k_d.$$

Things to ponder
Does it matter that we consider linear stretching forces instead of a non-linear form from (3.2)? How does the computation of μ_0, K to k_s, k_{al}, k_{ag} relation change when the non-linearity κ is involved?
Do the elastic coefficients depend on the number of mesh nodes? Hint: consider this first as a purely theoretical question and then practically for our case where we do not have completely regular triangular networks.

In-plane viscosity mode

To relate the viscosity coefficient k_{visc} to the biologically relevant membrane viscosity, often denoted by η_m, one can perform similar computations as we have done for the in-plane shear mode. Instead of applying the engineering strain to the regular triangular network, we apply a velocity field with a constant shear rate. Following this approach, Fedosov has obtained the relation [56, 158]:

$$\eta_m = \sqrt{3}(\gamma^T + \frac{1}{4}\gamma^C), \tag{4.13}$$

where the coefficients γ^T, γ^C appear in his definition of viscous forces:

$$\mathbf{F}_{visc}(A) = -\gamma^T \mathbf{v}_{AB} - \gamma^C (\mathbf{v}_{AB}, \mathbf{p}_{AB})\mathbf{p}_{AB}.$$

Comparing this expression with our formula for viscous forces (3.5) we see that he accounts for two viscous contributions: The second term is identical with our contribution and represents the projection of relative velocity onto the line AB. The first term defines force in the direction of the relative velocity. This extra contribution is necessary for stability of the DPD model presented in [56, 158], whereas in our IB-DC approach, this contribution is not needed.

To summarise, we make use of the relation (4.13) and state the following relation between the membrane viscosity and the spring network parameter:

$$\eta_m = \frac{\sqrt{3}}{4}k_{visc}.$$

There are different experimental ways to determine the membrane viscosity. Unfortunately, they give quite a wide range of viscosity values. Earlier works base their approach on a relaxation time t_c after large deformations of red blood cells caused by micropipette aspiration. During the recovery process after such deformation, the membrane viscosity dominates energy dissipation [54]. After measuring the relaxation time, one can assess the membrane viscosity through the relation $t_c = \eta_m/\mu_0$, as we already explained before the grey box at the end of Section 4.2.1. Here, μ_0 is the applied shear stress, resulting in values $\eta_m \approx 0.6\mu Ns/m$ reported in [93, 122].

Other types of experiments to determine the surface shear viscosity of the membrane were done in a rheoscope [188]. In these, individual erythrocytes were steadily tank-treading and the membrane viscosity was deduced from their dimensions and membrane rotational frequency. The reported values $\eta_m \approx 0.06\text{-}0.12\mu Ns/m$ are one order of magnitude lower than in the previous experiments.

Tether experiments reveal the upper bound of $0.005\mu Ns/m$ in [192]. Further, the diffusion constant of membrane-bound proteins can be used to calculate the membrane viscosity [163]. Using this approach, the values of RBC membrane viscosity have been reported in the range of $0.005\text{-}0.014\mu Ns/m$, obtained with various techniques [77, 190].

Out-of-plane bending mode

To relate the two bending parameters: k_b of the spring network model and k_c of the continuum model, we take a different approach than that from the in-plane contributions. We base our analysis on the bending energy of the spring network analogous to the Helfrich bending energy of the membrane introduced in Section 4.2.1.

In Appendix A.2, we show that our revisited definition of bending forces given by (3.8) is equivalent to the implementation of Kruger [107]. This allows us to use the results of [79, 107]. They derived the relation between the spring network parameter k_b and the continuum model parameter k_c from (4.3). The following relation holds for spherical shapes but is also widely used by others for general shapes:

$$k_b = \sqrt{3}k_c.$$

The value of k_c measured by micropipette aspiration is approximately $2 \times 10^{-19}Nm$ [53], while a review of several different measurements using various techniques gives a range $k_c = 1.15 \pm 0.9 \times 10^{-19}Nm$ [186].

Out-of-plane volume model

The biological background for the preservation of the cell volume lies in the osmotic equilibrium of the cell. The membrane is not completely impermeable, since it is responsible for the concentration equilibrium of osmotically active molecules inside the cell. The osmotic free energy [107] has the form

$$E_V = \frac{k_V}{2} \frac{V - V_0}{V_0},$$

with the biological value of the osmotic modulus $k_V = 7.23 \times 10^5 Jm^{-3}$. Our model does not capture this behavior and the volume preservation needs to be considered phenomenologically. Therefore, we have incorporated a mechanism to keep the volume almost unchanged.

In the model presented in [107], the author derives the biologically relevant values for volume preserving modulus $k_V = 7.23 \times 10^5 Jm^{-3}$ from the osmotic free energy. He claims, however, that the volume coefficient used in simulations is purely connected to the numerical properties of the computational model: the flow of fluid through the membrane. To compensate the undesired flow of fluid through the membrane - and thus to ensure volume preservation - he introduces the volume energy into the model and subsequent volume forces to keep the volume constant. The strength of these forces is however several orders of magnitude smaller than the biological value of k_V. A similar approach has been used by numerous other authors [56, 138, 189].

We adopt this approach as well, so the volume coefficient is chosen purely to maintain the volume of the cell and to have the maximal deviation of the volume under 1% of the cell volume in the relaxed state.

4.3   Calibration and validation experiments

Once we have a solid knowledge of linking the mechanical properties of the spring network models and the continuum models, we can look at practical implications. It must be repeated that almost all calculations in the previous sections have been performed for regular meshes with equilateral triangles. Similar computations could in principle also have been done for irregular triangular meshes but the relations between the parameters of the spring network models and the continuum models would become dependent on the local irregularities of the underlying triangular meshes.

Therefore, we have to hope that our triangular meshes are sufficiently similar to uniform meshes for the relations from the previous sections to hold.

Here we must be careful and not treat these relations as a ground truth. We should rather consider them as starting points for further fine-tuning of the values of elastic parameters for spring network meshes.

To this end, we employ experiments with real cells and we try to adapt those starting points in such a way that the computational model behaves as the real cells do. This fine-tuning is called the calibration of model parameters.

4.3.1 Stretching red blood cells

Even the slow physiological flows significantly distort the flexible red blood cells, making their ability to deform an essential feature of the mechanics. This ability ensures that the cells are capable of passing through narrow capillaries with diameters of less than half the cell diameter. To measure how flexible the cells truly are and how exactly they deform under controlled conditions, the cells have been examined in various experiments.

The earliest experiments used micrometer-scale pipettes to aspirate the cells [55]. Later, the aspiration techniques were refined [83] and more precise methods have been developed, such as measurements with optical tweezers [131], adhered magnetic bead cytometry [160] or microrheometry based on thermal fluctuations of cell shape [148]. In the following, we show how the optical tweezers experiment can be performed computationally and used to calibrate the elastic coefficients of the model.

In this experiment, two silica beads are attached to opposite sides of the cell rim, Figure 4.7. One of them is held in place and the other is pulled away using optical laser tweezers. The purpose of the silica beads is to be the laser targets.

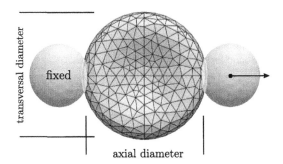

FIGURE 4.7: Principle of optical tweezers experiment with stretching of red blood cells.

The cell responds to this manipulation by stretching in the axial direction and contracting in the transversal direction. When stabilised, these two diameters are measured and paired up with the value of the applied force. The experiment is repeated several times with different forces and also with different cells, because we cannot expect them to behave exactly uniformly without some variation, Figure 4.8. The curves in the figure contain points that have been obtained by averaging the measurements of several cells. The error bars show the variance of the data.

The second part of this experiment is to release the silica beads and observe the relaxation to the original shape - both its duration and the transient shapes and non-linear evolution of the diameters.

To re-create the experiment in simulation, we do not have to keep the silica beads. Our *computational laser* is not going to hurt the cells and thus can be applied directly. Directly, but where? The diameter of the contact area of the silica beads is estimated to be 2 μm [131]. Therefore we want to apply force to the nodes around such diameter. We allow small deviation at both sides of this imaginary cell cut, since otherwise we would have only very few nodes directly on the cut circumference. Also, in order not to break the symmetry, we try to have the same number of nodes on both sides.

Following the previous guidelines, we have selected two groups of mesh points, together about 8% of all points. The first group has contained the points that lie on a (non-circular) ring and have the x-coordinate around 2-5% of the cell diameter. In the second group, there have been nodes that lie on the opposite ring and have the x-coordinate around 95-98% of the cell diameter.

```
# selection of particles for stretching
rightStretchedParticles = list()
leftStretchedParticles = list()
for i in cell.mesh.points:
    pos = (i.get_pos()[0]-cell.get_origin()[0])/resize
    if (pos >= xBoundMinR and pos <= xBoundMaxR):
        rightStretchedParticles.append(i)
    if (pos <= -xBoundMinL and pos >= -xBoundMaxL):
        leftStretchedParticles.append(i)
```

Things to ponder
Can we just take nodes whose x-coordinate is less than 5% or more than 95% of the cell diameter? Why or why not?

We have used the diameter of a biconcave red blood cell, $d = 7.82\mu m$ and confirmed that the contact diameter corresponds to the value reported in the literature. The total applied external force was then equally divided among these nodes.

The cell with a given set of five elastic parameters was then immersed in a stationary fluid. The external force has led to extension in the axial direction and to contraction in the transverse direction. When the object has achieved an equilibrium, we have measured the axial and transverse diameter. The same experiment was repeated for different applied forces and resulted in one force - displacement curve. The steps were then repeated for the next set of five elastic parameters and all resulting curves were compared to the experimental data.

Where did the sets of elastic parameters come from? The starting point is the theory of the membrane mechanics that gives us relations between the biological elastic moduli and model elastic parameters. Using these and the experimentally measured values of biological elastic moduli, we arrive at an initial set of elastic parameters $k_s = 0.0127$, $k_b = 0.0002$, $k_{al} = 0.0254$, $k_{ag} = 0.5$, $k_v = 0.9$ (see Appendix F.2). When we use them, we get a curve shown in Figure 4.8 (a). This is not ideal, but we need to remember that the coefficients were derived for a planar mesh with equilateral triangles. Our mesh is reasonably regular, but the triangles are not equilateral and of course, the mesh lies on a curved surface and not in a plane.

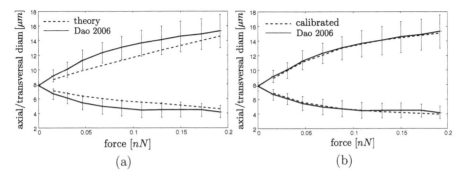

(a) (b)

FIGURE 4.8: Comparison of computational and experimental results from an optical tweezers stretching experiment. Experimental data from [40]. (a) Elastic coefficients as calculated from theory (under the assumption of having a planar mesh of equilateral triangles). (b) A slightly different set of coefficients.

Note, that a change of some of the parameters ($k_s = 0.006$, $k_b = 0.008$, $k_{al} = 0.001$, $k_{ag} = 0.5$, $k_v = 0.9$) gives a much better fit depicted in Figure 4.8 (b). Therefore, what is needed is a calibration of the elastic parameters, to find values close to the theoretically predicted values, for which the two curves, one for simulated data and one for experimental data, are comparable. Well, but how does one compare two curves?

Ideally, the best fit is when the two curves overlap. But is this really the ideal solution? We must realise that the points on the experimental curve were obtained by averaging values for several cells. So it could be possible that there is no single cell in the experiment that was actually prolonged to the value represented by one point on the experimental curve. It could just be a coincidence that this value was obtained by averaging different values.

The important information comes from the error bars in Figure 4.9. They show the variance of the data and it is reasonable to request that the simulation curve lies within these error bars. The fit of the simulation data to the

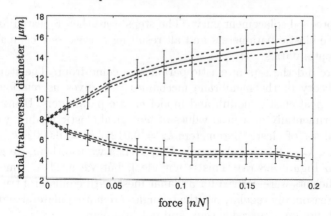

FIGURE 4.9: Experimental data from [40] (solid lines) with large error bars. For fitting the simulated curve within experimental data, the smaller region is indicated by dashed lines that lie within 25% of the error bars.

experimental data can be quantified by, e.g. defining an error function:

$$\sum_{1}^{10}((s_i^a - e_i^a)^2 + (s_i^t - e_i^t)^2),$$

where s^a and e^a are final simulated and experimental axial diameters, and s^t and e^t are final simulated and experimental transversal diameters. The sum goes through the experimentally available data, i.e. each index i corresponds to a different applied force. Such an error function is a non-negative function attaining its minimum just when the experimental and simulated data overlap.

At this point it is important to say that we do not aim at total minimisation of the error function. For us it is ok if the simulated curve lies within the error bars although the closer, the better. To get an idea about the validity range of the error function, let us compute the worst-case-scenario values.

By worst-case we mean curves at the minimal or maximal values of the error bars. Table 4.1 shows that even with the error function value 9 for transversal and 30 for axial curve, we are still within the error bars. Of course, these extremal values are not representative, so at this stage we could set a threshold of 1/4 of the error bar for the set of coefficients to be acceptable, which leads to a value of 0.56 for transversal curve and 1.89 for axial curves.

Stretching a cell using optical tweezers is certainly not the only thing experimentalists can do to investigate the elastic properties of cells. Laser can be used to stretch the cell without the need to use the silica beads [121], and there are many types of biological experiments where mechanical deformations can be observed. If a computational scientist can reproduce the experiment in a computer simulation, he or she can use the results to build confidence in the model - or, at least in a part of it. Let us look at a few other examples.

tolerance	Error function			
	trans min	trans max	axial min	axial max
error bar	9.01	9.16	30.25	27.80
0.24 error bar	0.56	0.57	1.89	1.74

TABLE 4.1: Error function values for worst-case scenario and thresholded case.

4.3.2 Couette/shear flow

Couette flow is shear flow between two parallel surfaces that move relative to one another. In practice, this means either one of them is stationary and the other moving or two plates moving with the same velocity in opposite directions.

Velocity

Suppose that the distance of the two (infinite) moving walls is h, the bottom wall is stationary and the top wall is moving with constant velocity $2v_0$ in the x-direction, as depicted in Figure 4.10 (a). We are interested in the velocity profile $\mathbf{v}$ between the walls. We assume that the only non-zero component of the fluid velocity field $\mathbf{v}$ will be in the x-direction and we denote this component by $v(y) = \mathbf{v}_x(x, y, z)$. There is no external pressure applied, and due to infinite walls we do not have pressure gradients. In this simple case, Navier-Stokes equations simplify to

$$\frac{d^2 v(y)}{dy^2} = 0,$$

where y is the spatial coordinate normal to the walls. With the boundary conditions $v(0) = 0$ and $v(h) = 2v_0$ we obtain an exact analytic solution:

$$v(y) = 2v_0 \frac{y}{h}.$$

Note that the first derivative of this velocity is constant and thus the velocity has a straight-line profile.

In case of two plates moving in opposite directions, Figure 4.10 (b), we also have a straight-line profile, with $v(h/2) = 0$. In this case, the relation for the exact solution is $v(y) = (v_0 - (-v_0))\frac{y}{h} = 2v_0 \frac{y}{h}$.

This setting is especially useful for the investigation of effects of shear on cells. If placed in the center of Couette flow, the cell experiences the shear stress but remains stationary (with respect to the x-direction), meaning that a small simulation box can be used.

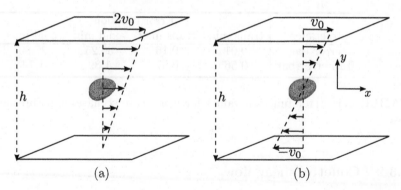

FIGURE 4.10: In Couette flow, fluid velocity is linear with respect to the y-coordinate. (a) The top wall moves with velocity $2v_0$ while the bottom wall remains static. The cell placed in the center starts to rotate and move to the right. (b) Two parallel walls move in opposite directions. The cell placed in the center rotates but remains at the same position.

Shear stress

The shear stress at a surface element located at height y above the plate, Figure 4.10 (a), is constant and given by

$$\tau(y) = \mu\frac{dv}{dy} = \mu\frac{2v_0}{h}. \qquad (4.14)$$

We see that it is directly proportional to the wall velocity and inversely proportional to the distance between plates.

Red blood cell in shear flow

Red blood cells exhibit rich behavioral patterns in a shear flow. Typically, an RBC exposed to a shear flow may elongate and align itself at a constant angle with respect to a flow. Under certain flow conditions, it may tumble or exhibit a tank-treading motion of the membrane or both, depending on the shear rate [138]. The biological laboratory experiments concerning the tumbling and tank-treading frequency have been reported, e.g. in [65, 188].

Shear flow can be simulated easily. An example computational domain can be a cubic box with dimensions $20 \times 20 \times 20\mu m^3$. The shear flow is generated by setting the constant horizontal velocity v_0 and $-v_0$ at the top and bottom boundaries of the channel, see Figure 4.10. In this setting with an empty channel, the velocity field has zero y and z components and the horizontal x component linearly decreases from the value v_0 at the top boundary to value $-v_0$ at the bottom boundary. This means that the shear rate $\dot{\gamma}$ is constant over the whole channel and equals

$$\dot{\gamma} = \frac{2v_0}{h},$$ (4.15)

where the height of the channel is denoted by h.

Shear stress vs. shear rate

Roughly speaking, *shear stress* in a two-dimensional case tells us how much shearing force in axial direction is applied per unit length in the transversal direction. When we are speaking of shear stress in fluid, the force is proportional not only to fluid velocity but also to fluid viscosity. For the simplified case of Couette flow, the shear stress in (4.14) is given by $\tau = \mu 2v_0/h$.

Shear rate, on the other hand, is a quantity used purely in connection with fluids and depends only on the fluid velocity, without an apparent connection to forces. Shear rate quantifies how fast the axial velocity changes when an observation point is moving in the transverse direction. So from (4.15) we have $\dot{\gamma} = 2v_0/h$.

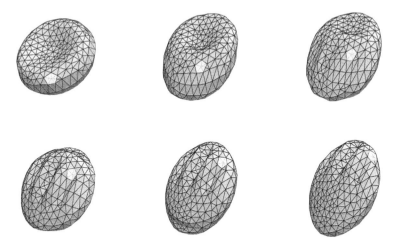

FIGURE 4.11: Deformation of the cell membrane during tank-treading motion under shear rate. One specific mesh point is highlighted in six time instances.

We have placed one cell in the middle of the channel. The simulation has shown that a red blood cell in a shear flow with certain wall velocities exhibits tumbling motion. At higher velocities this motion becomes tank-treading, which corresponds to previously presented results [158]. During the tumbling motion the cell rotates as a whole, while during the tank-treading motion the cell leans slightly and its membrane begins to rotate around the interior of the cell.

The speed of the rotation during the tumbling and tank-treading depends on the shear rate. This dependence has been shown by measuring the tank-treading frequency of live cells, and the data are available in [65, 158, 188].

To reproduce these experiments, we have used the density of fluid $1050 kg\,m^{-3}$ and viscosity $5Pa\,s$. These values correspond to biological solutions of dextran that is typically used in experiments [65, 188]. Snapshots of a tank-treading cell are depicted in Figure 4.11. From these snapshots we can see that the membrane rotates around the inner part of the cell and the shape changes from the relaxed biconcave shape into ellipsoid-like shape that does not change much.

During the simulation, coordinates of the mesh points are recorded so that the rotation frequency may be determined. In Figure 4.12, the experimental results are presented together with results obtained with the computational model. In this simulation, the elastic coefficients from Section 4.3.1 were used with the viscosity coefficient $k_{visc} = 0$. In this setup, the computational results show approximately 20% overshoot of the model compared to the biological data.

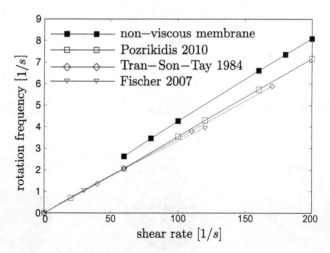

FIGURE 4.12: Rotation frequency for the original model (black solid squares) and experimental data (other marks) taken from [65, 158, 188]. Results from the original model are approximately 20% higher than experimental data.

In order to explain why we observe such an overshoot, we need to consider the following. The tank-treading motion of the cell introduces changes in the shape of the membrane. If any mechanism decreases the rate of these changes, it will decrease the rotational frequency and thus reduce the overshoot. Membrane viscosity is a property of the material that penalises fast changes of the shape and has exactly this desired effect.

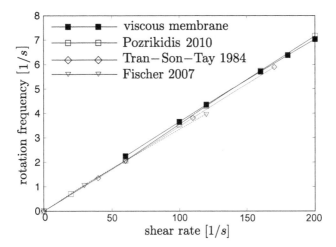

FIGURE 4.13: Rotation frequency for adjusted model which now also includes the viscoelastic modulus (black solid squares) and experimental data (other marks) taken from [65, 158, 188]. The model now gives results that conform to the experimental data.

Identical experiments performed with viscosity included in the model show a decrease in the rotational frequency. For calibration purposes, we have performed several simulations with different values of k_{visc}, ranging from 0 to 2.5. We have identified $k_{visc} = 1.5$ as the optimal value, with which we have obtained the results presented in Figure 4.13. We can see that the rotational movement of the cell has slowed down and the frequency fits the experimental data well.

4.3.3 Poiseuille flow and parachute shapes

Homogeneous fluid flow in a pipe is characterised by its parabolic profile and called Poiseuille flow. Normally, there is a pressure drop across the pipe, denoted by ΔP, which can be expressed as

$$\Delta P = \frac{8\mu LQ}{\pi R^4},\tag{4.16}$$

where L is the length of the pipe, R its inner radius, Q the volumetric flow rate (how much fluid flows through the fixed cross section during a unit time period) and μ the dynamic viscosity of the fluid.

Velocity

With a given volumetric flow rate, static distribution of the velocity profile develops with the following explicit expression, depending on r, the distance from the axis of the pipe

$$v(r) = \frac{\Delta P(R^2 - r^2)}{4\mu L} = \frac{2Q(R^2 - r^2)}{\pi R^4} \qquad (4.17)$$

with maximal value of the velocity for position on the axis of the pipe, that is for $r = 0$,

$$v_{max} = \frac{2Q}{\pi R^2}.$$

The position on the boundary of the pipe corresponds to $r = R$ and we directly see that the no-slip condition on the boundary is satisfied.

We need to compute the characteristics of the developed flow for given inflow-velocity v_{in}. In fact, we can easily compute the volumetric flow rate. Given v_{in} over a circular surface with the area $A = \pi R^2$, the volumetric flow rate is equal to

$$Q = v_{in} A = v_{in} \pi R^2.$$

Using this expression in (4.17) we get

$$v(r) = \frac{2Q(R^2 - r^2)}{\pi R^4} = \frac{2v_{in}(R^2 - r^2)}{R^2} \qquad (4.18)$$

with maximal value of the velocity for $r = 0$:

$$v_{max} = 2v_{in}.$$

This expression gives us an idea what v_{in} should be in order to develop a parabolic flow with a given maximal velocity in the middle of the pipe.

Shear stress

We know that the shear stress at a surface element parallel to the flat plate at the point in height y above the plate is given by

$$\tau(y) = \mu \frac{\partial v}{\partial y},$$

where μ is the dynamic viscosity of the fluid and v is the velocity of the fluid. The wall shear stress is then computed as

$$\tau_w = \tau(y = 0) = \mu \left. \frac{\partial v}{\partial y} \right|_{y=0}.$$

Replacing r in (4.18) by $R - y$ we get the expression for the shear stress:

$$\tau(y) = \mu \frac{\partial v}{\partial y} = \mu \frac{\partial}{\partial y} \left(\frac{2v_{in}(2Ry - y^2)}{R^2} \right) = \frac{2\mu v_{in}(2R - 2y)}{R^2}.$$

and finally, for wall shear stress:

$$\tau_w = \frac{4\mu v_{in}}{R}.$$

Red blood cell in Poisseuille flow

In [187], they perform experiments in a very narrow channel, where the cells deform to a parachute shape, see Figure 4.14. The experiments focus on the start-up dynamics so the model can be tested against dynamic data. Again, such experiments are well-suited to reconstruct *in-silico* (as also done in [60, 107]), since the flow conditions are given and narrow straight channels can be easily simulated.

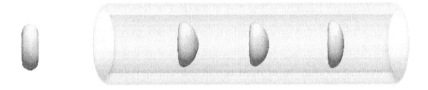

FIGURE 4.14: Snapshots of a cell forming a parachute-like shape similar to biological experiments performed in [187].

4.3.4 Other types of experiments in flow in confined regions

Microfluidics has been extensively used for cell manipulation. At the beginning of Chapter 6, we talk about applications of micro-flows in the processing of individual cells, where the cells are being manipulated by flow of surrounding fluid.

Deformation of cells in microfluidic devices can be caused by various phenomena. In flows with high cell density, the cell-cell interactions are the main cause of deformations. In dilute suspensions, the cell-cell encounters are rare and a cell deforms under the influence of the flow or the channel walls.

For the analysis of mechanical properties of individual cells, there are numerous techniques involving confined flows. Here, we make a distinction between those involving no contact with walls and those that allow cells to touch the channel boundaries. The reason for this is purely from the modeling perspective: If a cell comes into contact with a channel wall, the friction between the membrane and the wall surface affects the cell movement. This friction is another phenomenon that must be included in the model. This brings more complexity to the model and therefore, the experiments without cell-wall interaction are more suitable for assessing the membrane mechanics.

Experiments without cell-wall contact

Cells are flexible and when they are subjected to a shear stress, they deform. The actual deformation depends on the shear rate the cell is exposed to. To create a sufficiently large shear rate, a constriction within the channel has been frequently used. The size of the constriction must naturally be larger than the size of the cell in case we want no contact with the walls. Depending on the size of the constriction and the position of the flowing cells entering the constriction, the cells start to exhibit various types of behavior. They may tumble, tank-tread, or, if they enter the constriction *head-on*, they adopt a parachute-like shape.

In [198], they perform an extensive analysis of cell entering a constriction. They state that the cells exhibit five different modes according to position of the cell entering the constriction:

Stretching - Elongation in the direction of flow, without rotation

Tumbling - Rotation around the major axis perpendicular to the direction of flow

Twisting - Rotation around the major axis parallel to the flow direction

Rolling - Rotation around the minor axis perpendicular to the direction of flow

Complex - All other motions

The data provided in this work include information from all modes such as the prolongation of cells during the stretching mode, tumbling frequency in tumbling mode and radial velocity of cells in rolling mode. Twisting mode is more difficult to observe because the cells were visualised only along one direction. The available visual data allow to quantify the twisting by introducing the relative magnitude of rotation characterised by the change in the projected aspect ratio.

Since the fluid conditions are well defined by providing a constant flow rate of the cell suspension, such an experimental setup can be modeled computationally and this experiment is thus suitable for validation of the model.

Another type of experiment suitable for assessing the cell deformation index has been described in [162]. In it the cells pass a sequence of three hyperbolic converging microchannels. One of the three sections is depicted in Figure 4.15. In the narrowest part of the channel, the cell is most deformed and once it reaches the wide portion of the next section, it relaxes back to the biconcave discoid shape. In the process, the deformation index can be measured.

For simulation, the critical region of this experiment is where the narrow part suddenly widens. There is a rapid change of fluid and cell velocity and fine steps are needed to resolve it correctly. The work [162] has observed both RBCs and WBCs in this channel and - as expected - found that the white blood cells are significantly stiffer than erythrocytes.

Deformation index

The deformation index (DI) is calculated as

$$DI = \frac{a-b}{a+b},$$

where a is the major axis and b is the minor axis of the red blood cell (or another object) as seen in a 2D image.

Clearly this is an imperfect characteristic, since it only describes a 2D projection of a 3D object. We could certainly get two objects with different deformations resulting in the same DI. It is used because it utilises measurements that can be obtained automatically from image processing of videos of experiments with many cells. Comparing the actual deformation would be much more complicated.

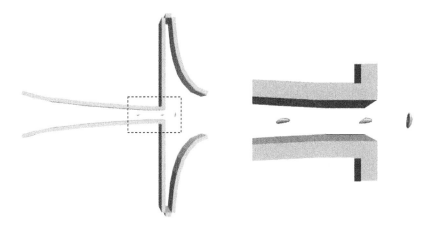

FIGURE 4.15: Snapshots of a cell passing through one of several identical parts of a hyperbolic channel similar to biological experiments performed in [162].

The work [154] has proposed a microfluidic device that can perform both RBC separation and deformability analysis. The deformability is also characterised by the DI.

Experiments including cell-wall contact

When the constriction has smaller dimensions than the cell, the cell comes into contact with walls. In Figure 4.16 a cell enters a narrow gap. It is being deformed and depending on the stiffness of the membrane, it takes some time to enter the constriction. Such an experiment can easily be set up, however we must also bear in mind that the friction between the cell membrane and the wall plays a role here.

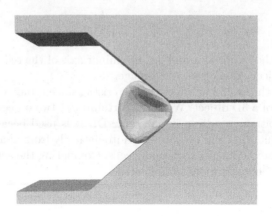

FIGURE 4.16: Cell entering a constriction with cell-wall contact.

The study [2] observes red blood cell deformation in such constriction and provides both suspension-level and single-cell measurements. On the single-cell scale, they focus on the actual shapes and provide a more detailed cell characteristic compared to simple DI.

4.3.5   Experimental data for elasticity of other blood cells

White blood cells

White blood cells have an internal viscosity many times higher than the red blood cells and thus do not deform nearly as much under the same flow conditions, as shown in [162]. Unlike the red blood cells, they also contain a nucleus and this contributes to their lower deformability. There are various types of WBCs, so the elastic and viscous properties vary among them, but to give at least some notion we mention the following two studies.

In [151] elastic properties of individual leukocytes in their passive state were studied by the micropipette aspiration technique. Their passive elastic rigidity (PER) defined as steady-state deformation normalised for the pipette radius divided by stress was measured. For healthy lymphocytes, $PER = 349.7 \pm 125.9 \mu N/m$ and for healthy granulocytes, $PER = 226.5 \pm 86.7 \mu N/m$ which is significantly larger than the shear modulus and area compression modulus measured for RBCs. The values reported for leukemic WBCs are about half of those for healthy WBCs.

In [83], a different deformability measurement technique was proposed. In principle, it is equivalent to whole cell micropipette aspiration, but involves simpler operation, involves less specialised equipment and requires less technical skill. Single cells are flown through a microfluidic channel and deformed through a series of funnel-shaped constrictions. The constriction openings are sized to create a temporary seal with each cell as it passes through the constriction. This way they replicate the interaction with the micropipette opening. The study indicated the threshold pressures and deformation indices for various types of WBCs as they pass the openings. Also cortical tension is measured.

Platelets

Platelets are smaller than red blood cells and have a vital role under life-threatening conditions. Similarly to RBCs they do not contain nuclei. During their inactive state they are practically non-deformable and have a discoid shape with a diameter of 2-4μm. When they are active - forming blood clots to prevent blood loss during injuries - they change their shape very rapidly and take an irregular branched spread form [38]. Their adhesive dynamics was studied in, e.g. [134]. In Section 6.8, we mention how wall roughness may influence their near-wall behavior.

Circulating tumor cells

We have already mentioned the [151] study, which compared healthy and cancerous cells. Similarly, [11] measures deformability differences between tumor cells and blood cells. To assess the differences, they have used a U-shaped resonator and have compared passage times of different cells through the constriction of a specific length. Multiple scatter plots are presented of passage time vs. buoyant mass or vs. volume of cells. In [81], they analyse cells at throughputs, which are orders of magnitude larger than previously reported using biophysical flow cytometers and single-cell mechanics tools. Two carefully aligned flows from opposite directions are collided and a cell coming in from one of them is flushed to the side. Just before that happens, while it is still at the *crossroads*, its deformability is measured as the ratio of its major to minor axis. Using this approach, it is possible to quickly assess deformability of a large number of leukocytes and malignant cells and accurately predict disease state in patients with cancer and immune activation with a sensitivity of 91% and a specificity of 86%. Similarly to [151], they report that benign cells have lower deformability than the cancerous ones. They state the hypothesis that the increased deformability of tumor cells may contribute to the capability of these cells to create metastases. Note though that the circulating tumor cells, while more deformable than WBCs, are still significantly stiffer than RBCs.

In [98], they present a detailed experimental analysis of time evolution of cell position during the transit of cell through the channel, similar to that in Figure 4.16. Several scatter plots are presented such as elongation index vs. cell size, transit velocity vs. elongation index and entry time vs. elongation index.

4.4   Issues with biological data

Several times in this book, we have referred to biological experiments with red blood cells, considering them the gold standard, against which the models should be fitted and compared. Such comparisons, while extremely useful and unquestioningly necessary, bring with themselves a whole new set of issues. Here we mention some of them to hint at possible complications during the validation of the model.

4.4.1   Limitations of single-cell calibration experiments

How would an ideal validation experiment look? For example, for the membrane shear modulus, it would mean to cut out a small rectangular portion of the membrane, carefully flatten it out, keep its biomechanical properties intact in the process, and then stretch it in two opposite directions with known force. Measure the dimensions of the stretched sheet and derive the shear modulus. Unfortunately, such an experiment is (as of now) not possible.

One of the first experiments that the modelers relied on, was the micropipette aspiration experiment. Their limitation was that to measure a local parameter - the membrane shear modulus - they involved the whole cell, a significant portion of which has been aspirated into a pipette and the measured deformation fitted to theoretical expectations.

Nowadays, one of the most widely used experiments - the stretching of RBC using optical tweezers (discussed in Section 4.3.1) - also measures the response of the whole cell. And even if we disregard this issue, in [45] it has been discussed that when using a continuum description of the RBC membrane, the only constitutive law able to match well the wide variety of experimental data is the Skalak law [173]. As a consequence, the shear modulus as examined in, e.g. [131], which represents the Yeoh law is not the true shear modulus of the RBC membrane. In [45], it has also been argued that the strain-softening models, such as the neo-Hookean and Evans laws, overestimate the erythrocyte shear modulus. Nevertheless, the data from the optical tweezers experiment continue to be used for validation of various RBC membrane models, and not only for continuum models, for which they were originally intended, but also for mesh-based models such as the one described in this book once the relationship to the continuous parameters is found.

Another issue with the optical tweezers experiment, also mentioned in [56], is that it only measures two diameters: axial and transversal, as visible from a single observation angle. The cells might rotate slightly as they are being stretched and thus distort the transversal measurement. Moreover, the measurements do not take into account the way the cell deforms in the center at all. The introduction of two additional lengths is proposed in [172]. They are measured in the direction perpendicular to the plane of the RBC: the in-plane length, i.e. thickness of the cell, and the folding length, i.e. the depth of the dip at the center of the cell. Such experimental measurements could be more helpful to characterise the mechanics of the RBC membrane.

With these limitations in mind, we can still use the data to calibrate the model parameters, but we cannot treat them as absolute truths but rather as an approximations of the true values.

4.4.2 Replicating experimental setup in simulation

Suppose we have perfectly solved all the issues from the previous section and now we have a well-fitted cell model. Now we would like to use it and simulate a dynamical experiment with flow and many such cells. How do we set up a simulation with many cells that corresponds to the experiment?

Besides the mechanical properties of the cells, we need to have a proper model for the fluid and control the simulation setup. This means, for example, using the same flow rate as was used in the experiment. This is again a non-trivial task. Even in experiments that mechanically keep the flow rate constant, we may experience small fluctuations. The microfluidic cell-scale simulations typically do not simulate the whole device, just some critical parts, such as junctions, periodic blocks, etc. and at this scale, the fluctuations may be significant.

Also, if some other part of the device gets blocked, e.g. a cell gets stuck in one of 10 identical parallel microchannels that have a common inlet and outlet, the remaining 9 now experience a different flow rate - the total flow rate is not divided by 10 but just by 9. If we just simulate one of them and compare the results with video of one of them, we might not even be aware that some other channel was blocked and that our flow rate had changed. Similar issues may arise in periodic obstacle arrays.

Another issue is that the computational experiments have to be seeded. How to match the distribution of cells in the flow well? Typically, one lets the initial transients pass and only considers the subsequent observations but even so, we will never have exact match of positions, rotations, local velocities, cell variations, etc.

4.4.3 Need for image processing

Now suppose that we are reasonably sure that the biological and computational experiments are well matched. To check that the results match too, we need to extract the relevant information from a video recording of the experiment. This requires image processing, illustrated in Figure 4.17, which is a discipline of its own.

After a background is subtracted from all images, edges can be detected and a circle version of the Hough transformation used to determine the centers of cells. The centers can be used for cell tracking. Tracking means connecting the cell centers in subsequent images into tracks. This may be complicated

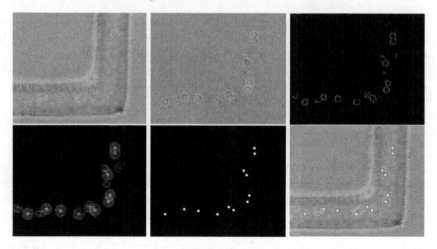

FIGURE 4.17: Steps in cell detection (from top left): original snapshot, background subtraction, edge detection, Hough transform for detection of centers, detected cell centers, original snapshot with detected cell centers. Experimental images from [127].

because when making the video recording, the focus is at a certain depth of the channel and cells that flow lower or higher may be blurry. That might be a reason why they are not detected and might be missing from the track.

Missing cells are not the only thing that complicates cell tracking. Another complication is when a cell passes over or under another cell or cells. This way two or more tracks join and information from previous steps has to be used to determine which cell is which once they separate. The goal is to obtain tracks of individual cells with the cell center positions and bounding boxes. From this information and frame rate, one can also determine cell velocity and angular velocity.

4.4.4   Validation of flow of many cells on a single-cell scale

Finally, suppose that the image processing went smoothly and we have a beautiful set of biological data that involves many cells in flow. While it may be relatively easy to compare single-cell experiments, such as the stretching experiments discussed in Section 4.3.1, which conveniently also include the cell measurements, it is not immediately clear how to compare the two flows of many cells. The flows obviously cannot by compared cell-by-cell, frame-by-frame. The individual trajectories, positions, rotations and velocities will not match exactly, because it is virtually impossible to seed all the cells exactly as they entered the simulated chamber, with exactly the same properties and spatial characteristics. The only other option is to do statistical comparison and a natural question is comparison of what?

There are two principal kinds of parameters, which can be used to compare a numerical simulation with a laboratory experiment. The first type helps us to do the comparison from static frames, where we can observe the position of cells in the microfluidic device or their inclination [9]. The second type can be obtained from a video or a sequence of frames, e.g. the velocity or rotation of the cells.

The work [10] uses discrete Fourier transform and the Kendall's tau rank correlation analysis to examine the rotations and angular speeds of cells. It appears that this approach can discern similarities and differences between types of flow. Another study [174] analyses selected characteristics such as cell orientation with respect to flow that can further be used for statistical comparisons of the flows using principal component analysis. Similar kinds of statistical comparison methods need to be developed to validate flows of many cells.

Chapter 5

Practical issues

5.1   Introduction

In the previous chapters, we introduced a model and looked at its verification and validation. In the process, we have silently assumed that we know how to get this model to work in a computer, but sometimes this might not be straightforward. Therefore, we now return to few practical issues, which might pose a problem.

This chapter is not meant to be read in a linear fashion, but rather as a collection of individual topics, from which the reader can choose, or even skip altogether. The topics involve the actual programming and while this is not a book on programming, we also want to mention a few general hints and insights that might be useful when implementing models.

In an ideal world, writing a program or a simulation script should involve three people: a person who comes up with the idea, a person who implements it and a person who tests it. The reasoning behind this is that if one of them does not think about a certain aspect of the problem, another one would catch it somewhere in the process.

As we all know, we do not live in an ideal world and chances are that you are on your own, thinking up your code, writing it and if there is enough time, doing some tests, too. Here we summarise some tips that are worth keeping in mind while doing so:

- **Write comments in your code.** Take notes. Work on documentation simultaneously as you write the code. Whatever works. This is both for you, to clarify your thoughts, to avoid mistakes and to be able to understand your own work once you try to return to it after some time (be it weeks, months or years) and also for others who can thus more easily understand, check and build on it. Think about how experimentalists work in labs. They have protocols to follow, they write lab journals to document the experiments they performed so that these can be replicated later or by someone else.

- **Keep it simple.** Break it into smaller parts. Such code is easier to debug, test, understand, reuse.

- **Test.** There is no way around it. Many people find it boring or an unproductive slowdown from more creative work, but it is an essential part of programming and making sure that you are not getting some mysterious new results, which are just errors in disguise. It might be interesting to know there are also people out there who write tests even before the actual implementation of the desired functionality. And if there is a bug fixed, consider writing a new unit test for it, so that the same situation does not repeat again. More on why the unit testing is very useful: [185].

- **Do not optimise too soon.** As Donald Knuth famously stated, optimising prematurely often leads to future trouble. Start with simple, even if slow or naïve codes that do what you need. Check that they truly do. Profile which parts take long. Consider if it is too long. Only then optimise.

- **Do not modify everything at once.** Take small steps, otherwise you end up with a big mess that takes much longer to fix.

- **Use existing solutions with judgement.** There is no point in re-inventing a wheel. The same way as most of us do not write our own operating systems or various applications, sometimes it makes sense to outsource those parts of our models that somebody has already done very well. For example throughout this book, we have cells immersed in fluid, which we have not coded ourselves and we rely on the lattice-Boltzmann implementation in ESPResSo. This is all fine and well as long as the outsourced code (and by extension library, module, programming language) is reliable and stable. Look for solutions that have been around for a while, so that they are no longer in the cannibalistic early evolutionary phases and have a potential to stay for a while: they have a reasonable user base and community of developers.

- **Try to find cases where you can verify computational results exactly.** Either by comparing with theory and analytical results or by comparing statistical outputs to experimental data. Also try to think what should happen in extreme cases. Compare that with what actually does happen in your code. This goes back to the verification we have already talked about in Section 4.1.1.

- **Be skeptical.** When you get results, both expected and unexpected, pause and think whether they are reasonable: check if they are correct at least to the order of magnitude, etc. Try to avoid confirmation bias. Expect failure. It is just an overhead for getting hits.

5.2 Periodicity of the simulation domain

In microfluidics, we are often looking at simulations of portions of long channels or of periodically repeating blocks. In these cases, it is often computationally advantageous not to simulate the whole thing, but a suitably selected portion instead. Think of a long channel. Instead of simulating it whole, cut it up into smaller pieces, as in Figure 5.1 and apply periodic boundary conditions.

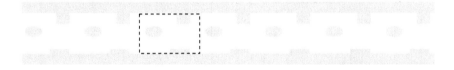

FIGURE 5.1: Long channel containing obstacles (top view) with periodically repeating blocks. One such block is indicated by the dashed line. Periodic boundary conditions may be applied on the left and right side of the dashed rectangle.

In general, the periodic boundary conditions are as follows: In the absence of any walls in a simulation box with dimensions $box_x \times box_y \times box_z$, the velocity $\mathbf{v}$ meets the conditions

$$\mathbf{v}(0, y, z) = \mathbf{v}(box_x, y, z) \qquad \forall y, z$$
$$\mathbf{v}(x, 0, z) = \mathbf{v}(x, box_y, z) \qquad \forall x, z$$
$$\mathbf{v}(x, y, 0) = \mathbf{v}(x, y, box_z) \qquad \forall x, y$$

Applying these conditions is both very useful and at times constricting. Let us discuss the usefulness here and the disadvantages in the next subsection.

Using these conditions, it is easy to simulate a part of a larger device with periodically repeating blocks. In this situation, the simulated part can be thought of as a moving window, because the cells exiting, e.g. in the positive *x*-direction, will enter the box again from the negative *x*-direction, e.g. if the simulation box has dimensions $50 \times 40 \times 30$ and a cell leaves it at a position [50, 24, 13], it can reenter at [0, 24, 13]. The same approach applies to the *y*- and *z*-coordinates. The advantage is that there is no need to delete the old object and create a new one (completely, with corresponding interactions), the same ones can be used. In ESPResSo, this is done using the *folded* commands.

Shifted periodicity and reseeding of cells

The periodic boundary conditions work very well for scenarios, which are indeed periodic. But what about situations where the periodicity is shifted or even absent?

In applications involving deterministic lateral displacement, we would need shifted periodicity. While possible to implement, it is much more complicated than the regular periodic boundary conditions. One workaround is to include some *buffer space* before the first row and after the second row of obstacles, e.g. as depicted in Figure 5.2. Only part of the simulation domain is then used for actual observations and data collection. This can be thought of as *spatial initialisation* (as opposed to *temporal initialisation*).

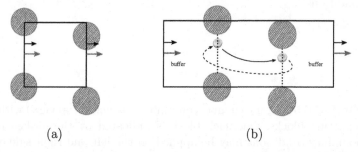

(a)   (b)

FIGURE 5.2: Simulated domains (thick black lines) with periodic boundary conditions within a periodic obstacle array (dashed circles). (a) The setting as depicted is useless because periodicity sets incorrect fluid velocities, for example a non-zero velocity inside an obstacle (black arrow within the dashed circle). (b) Using a sufficiently large buffer space before and after the repeating block, the velocity field adapts itself to maintain (almost exact) shifted boundary conditions. Flowing cells are reseeded back at the dotted line as indicated by the dashed arrow.

In such situations, we need to take care of reseeding of cells, i.e. remove them from the end of the observation window and place them at the correct position at the beginning of the observation window, Figure 5.2 (b). The same rules apply as when using periodicity: this kind of recycling is useful when the cells in the simulation are essentially *the same*. They may differ by their orientation with respect to the flow or by their current deformation, but they have the same resting shape, same size and same elastic properties. If this is the case, we can take the cell that leaves the simulation box on one end and place it at a respective location at the other end.

From here, it is just one more step to the situation with no periodicity at all. Consider an L-shaped channel depicted in Figure 5.3. This kind of channel may be used for examining connectors of microfluidic devices or optimising curve shapes in channels. The same principle may be used, cells can be re-seeded at appropriate flow locations, but additional care needs to be taken to rotate them, see example in Figure 5.3. The boundary conditions for the fluid should correspond to the parabolic profile of Poiseuille flow.

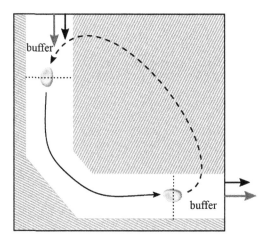

FIGURE 5.3: Reseeding of cells in an L-shaped channel. In addition to specifying proper position at the channel entry, rotation also has to be performed, in this case by 90 degrees.

5.3 Seeding of dense suspensions

When you are in the modeling business, sooner or later you start to come to terms with the fact that some things are not precise. That is not necessarily a bad thing, as long as we can get reasonably good solutions of the proper problems. It is certainly better than having precise solutions of wrong problems, no matter how detailed these problems or models are.

For some applications, it is desired to have many irregular objects (e.g. deformed randomly distributed cells) seeded in various domains. Obviously, one can find a precise solution to a wrong problem: e.g. achieve a dense regular seeding, Figure 5.4. Such seeding then requires a long transient time for the artificial regularity to vanish. The common convention is to require a particle with average flow velocity to circulate the geometry 10 times (using the periodic boundary conditions described in the previous section) before the actual simulation is started [197]. A discussion of how to properly do this, including the safety layer between pairs of cells, can be found in [107].

```
# generating regular seeding positions
cell_positions = list()
for k in range(0, 2):
    for l in range(0, 4):
        for m in range(0, 5):
            cell_positions.append([5.0+l*10, 4.0+m*3, 5.0+k*10])
```

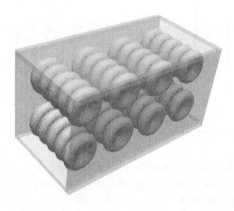

FIGURE 5.4: Regular seeding, Ht=28%.

It is also possible (at least in principle) to find a bad solution to the proper problem: e.g. create a dense seeding by deterministically specifying the positions and specifying the precise deformation of each cell. This approach certainly cannot be recommended as an actual solution, because it is extremely impractical. A better approach is to try to find a method that would give a reasonably good seeding even though it might not be achieved by completely physical steps.

Hematocrit
Hematocrit denoted by Ht is the ratio of the volume of red blood cells to the total volume of blood or cell suspension.

5.3.1   Random seeding

The obvious first choice is seeding the cells at random positions and giving them random rotation. While easy to do, this approach without any modifications has one major drawback. It is only suitable for very small volume fractions. For Ht > 10% it gets impractical due to the shape of the red blood cell. One can either use a code similar to the snipped presented here, where each RBC *reserves* space that corresponds to a circumscribed sphere and then later generates random rotation for the actual cell placement. Alternatively, one could place the cell and employ more sophisticated collision detection when evaluating another cell position and rotation. Random packing of bi concave discoids does not work nearly as well as random packings of spheres, see Figure 5.5.

```
# generating random seeding positions of cells
cell_positions = list()
trial_counter = 0
for k in range(0,n_cells):
    origin_ok = 0
    while origin_ok != 1 and trial_counter < max_no_of_trials:
        # generate random position in channel;
        ox = random.random() * (boxX - 2*rbc_radius) + rbc_radius
        oy = random.random() * (boxY - 2*rbc_radius - 2) + 1 + rbc_radius
        oz = random.random() * (boxZ - 2*rbc_radius - 2) + 1 + rbc_radius
        origin_ok = 1
        trial_counter += 1

        # check that it does not collide with other rbcs
        if origin_ok == 1:
            for i in range(0,k):
                dist = oif.vec_distance([ox, oy, oz], cell_positions[i])
                if dist < 2*rbc_radius:
                    origin_ok = 0
                    break

        # if everything was ok, remember origin
        if origin_ok == 1:
            cell_positions.append([ox,oy,oz])
```

It is possible to partially resolve the problem of large spaces between cells in random seeding by allowing some overlap of the cells, Figure 5.6. Obviously, this is an unphysical behavior - biological cells do not overlap - but if we could deal with the overlap in the initial transient phase of the simulation (think about it as a warm-up of the whole system using a repulsive potential), then the actual simulation of interest would start only after the initialisation is complete and the cells do not overlap anymore.

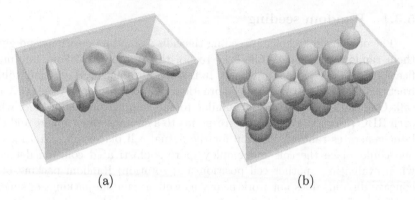

(a) (b)

FIGURE 5.5: Random seeding of RBCs and spheres. The volume of one RBC is the same as volume of one sphere. (a) Red blood cells, Ht (volume fraction) = 8.4%. (b) Spheres, volume fraction = 23.5%.

```
# check that generated origin does not collide with other rbc
# while allowing overlap
allowed_overlap = 0.3
if origin_ok == 1:
        for i in range(0,k):
                dist = oif.vec_distance([ox, oy, oz], cell_positions[i])
                if dist < (1.0 - allowed_overlap)*2*rbc_radius:
                    origin_ok = 0
                    break
```

This way, it is possible to achieve an RBC volume fraction of about 20% in a reasonably short time.

5.3.2 Cell growth

The actual problem with seeding lies in specifying the deformations of the individual cells. So why not use the same mechanism that is responsible for deformations and let it do the work also during initialisation? Small cells, e.g. half-diameter and thus one-eighth volume fraction, can be seeded at random in relaxed state and then grown to their proper size. The works [33, 125] have used this approach with cells that were rigid during the growth phase. In [107], the growing particles were elastic and the absence of ambient fluid was compensated by adding an artificial repulsive force that ensured that the opposite concave parts of the membrane did not intersect.

The cell-cell interactions can ensure that the membranes of neighboring cells do not overlap but rather deform, when the cells get too close. While this idea is sound, it does not work well in a system where the individual bonds

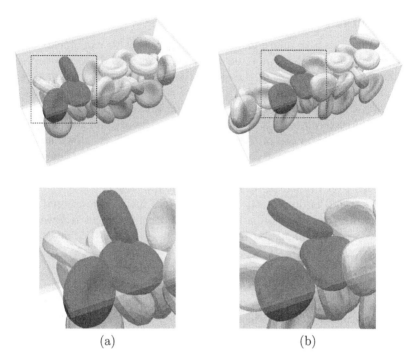

FIGURE 5.6: Random seeding of RBCs with initial overlap allowed, Ht = 19.6%. (a) Initial positions with overlap. (b) Membrane collision interaction resolved overlaps.

among surface nodes specify the elastic properties, since these would have to be repeatedly re-defined.

This issue poses less of a problem if we re-specify just the global interactions responsible for conservation of surface or volume, as it was done in [101]. This means, we could technically seed spherical objects with desired surface and then decrease (in small steps) their volume to the cell volume. Alternatively, we could seed spheres with the desired volume and gradually increase their surface. The second approach is more suitable because it allows more objects in the given simulation box. However, both are problematic, since the resting shape of both types of resulting cells is a sphere and not a biconcave discoid.

Note that in principle, the improvement using initial overlap can also be used in this kind of seeding. With such overlap, it is possible to achieve up to 45% Ht.

5.3.3 Free fall

Another idea is to take advantage of the fact that we can quickly and easily seed simulations that are not too dense. We can then do a two-step seeding. In the first step, we expand the simulation box along the largest face of the original box (e.g. if the original was $40 \times 20 \times 20$, the expanded box will be $40 \times 20 \times 40$). We randomly seed this larger box and then we apply artificial external force to all cells that drives them to the original box, Figure 5.7. If the extension sits on top of the original box, the cells fall down as if dragged by gravity, hence the name *free fall* for this approach. It is of course, possible to combine this with the previously mentioned idea and allow some initial overlap in order to increase the final volume fraction.

The free fall is done until all the cells are inside the original region (in our case, until the z-coordinate of their upper-most point is lower than the z-dimension of the simulated box.

```
# fall part of the free fall seeding
checkZ = False
for i in range(1, maxCycle):
    system.integrator.run(steps=500)
    print "time: ", str(i*system.time_step)
    # check if everything is in lower box
    checkZ = True
    for rbc in enumerate(rbcs):
            maxZ = rbc.get_pos_bounds[5]
        if maxZ > boxZ-boundary_thickness:
            checkZ = False
    if checkZ:
        break
for id, rbc in enumerate(rbcs):
    rbc.output_mesh_points(file_name="cell" + str(id) + ".dat")
```

Most likely the cells will be pushed against one of the walls when we save their positions. We then load these positions into a second simulation, in which the fluid is stationary. In this second part, we use the original box and apply external force in random direction to each cell. This external force together with repulsive cell-cell interactions ensures that the cells distribute evenly over the whole simulation chamber even if there are obstacles present, Figure 5.8. The advantage of this random shaking approach is that we can repeat the second step several times to get different seedings from one free fall.

```
# creating the template for RBCs
type = oif.OifCellType(nodes_file="input/rbc374nodes.dat", \
triangles_file="input/rbc374triangles.dat", check_orientation=False, \
system=system, ks=rbc_ks, kb=rbc_kb, kal=rbc_kal, kag=rbc_kag, \
kv=rbc_kv, normal=True, resize=[rbc_radius, rbc_radius, rbc_radius])
```

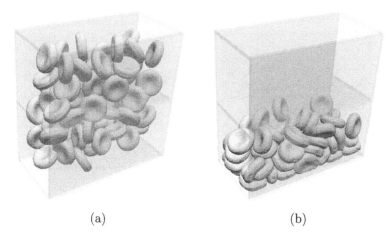

(a)   (b)

FIGURE 5.7: Using free fall to initialise a dense suspension. (a) A simulation box of double size is seeded and artificial gravity is applied. (b) Once all cells fall into the original box, their positions are saved.

```
# creating the RBCs using stored nodes files
rbcs = list()
for id in range(0, n_cells) :
    cell_rbc = oif.OifCell(cell_type=type, particle_type=id, \
    origin=[0.0, 0.0, 0.0], particle_mass=0.5)
    # set node positions
    cell_rbc.set_mesh_points("cell" + str(id) + ".dat")
    rbcs.append(cell_rbc)

# preparing random external forces for the shake phase of free fall seeding
for id, rbc in enumerate(rbcs):
    rbc.set_force([random.random()*0.001-0.0005, \
    random.random()*0.001-0.0005, random.random()*0.001-0.0005])
```

Possible issues and extensions: Note the stopping criterion for the first step of this seeding: the simulation runs until all cells move into the original box. Even though this sounds fairly inconspicuous, in practice it might lead to an unexpectedly long wait. A typical situation is that most of the cells get to the original box fairly quickly and then the last one or the last few take a long time. To avoid this wait, it is reasonable to initially seed a few more cells than needed and then stop the free fall once the required number of cells make it into the original box.

Another improvement might be to use not just a few more cells in the free fall step, but about 1.5-2 times as many and then randomly select the desired

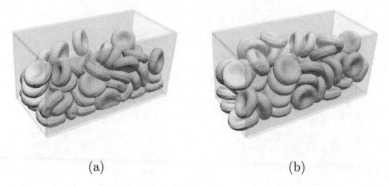

(a)   (b)

FIGURE 5.8: Using free fall to initialise a dense suspension. (a) Cell positions obtained from free fall are loaded into the desired box and random forces are applied to each cell to *shake* the suspension. Cell-cell and cell-wall interactions also contribute to the process. (b) Final seeding positions, Ht = 43%.

number of them for the shaking phase. This will allow more variation in the initial configuration when one wants to have many different random seedings in the same configuration.

The cell membrane elasticity is not physically accurate in these seeding simulations. Typically, the cells need to be stiffer so that they survive being squeezed in the crowd against the wall. The (already non-physical) repulsive cell-wall interactions need to be stronger for the same reason. We do not need to worry about this, since the seeding output are just positions of membrane nodes and these are later loaded as input in the actual simulation of interest, where the cells and interactions have proper parameters.

A natural extension is also the following: why not use something that can already do the free fall of objects quickly? Computer games are known for having strong physical engines at their cores, capable of collision detection and resolving interactions. Examples of such engines are Bullet Physics Library [36] (with Blender Creation Suite [66]) or Open Dynamics Engine [176].

It is not necessary to use elastic objects for the seeding (and some engines might not even have the capabilities to perform elastic collisions). We can imagine pouring rigid objects into the box and letting gravity do the work. Objects will not overlap, their positions will be saved in the desired format and then loaded into a simulation with elasticity.

Things to ponder

Can you come up with other ideas on how to seed a dense suspension?

5.4 Discretisation

Numerical implementations often involve discretisation of space or time or both. This discretisation necessarily introduces errors. Even more so when different parts of the model have their own discretisation: i.e. fluid uses a regular rectangular grid and elastic objects use reasonably regular triangular meshes. Obviously, there is also the time discretisation of the whole system. These all need to correspond to each other (e.g. the two spatial discretisations via the friction coefficient described in Section 3.5) in order for the model to work properly.

Speed of sound
In the air, the sound propagates with the speed approximately $343 m/s$, with the exact value depending on the air humidity, density and other factors.

In the lattice-Boltzmann method, a three-dimensional lattice is used to model fluid flow. Here, a similar notion, *lattice speed of sound*, is defined, often denoted by c_s that represents how fast any information can travel within the lattice. This speed is always given in units $\Delta x/\Delta t$ because the information can move only along the edges or diagonals of the lattice. The concrete value of c_s depends on the implementation of the lattice-Boltzman method. For the D3Q19 version, it is $c_s = 1/\sqrt{3}$.

Lattice Mach number
Mach number as used in fluid dynamics is the ratio of flow velocity to the local speed of sound. For an aircraft, it is its ground speed divided by the speed of sound.

For the lattice-Boltzmann method, the *lattice Mach number* denoted by Ma follows the same concept using the lattice speed of sound

$$Ma = u/c_s,$$

where u is the fluid velocity.

5.4.1 Triangular mesh vs. fluid lattice

If we use a discretisation with too few membrane nodes, the large cell membrane deformations cannot be resolved properly. But if too many nodes are used, it increases the computational cost, especially if there are many cells in the simulation. One has to look for a suitable middle ground. Once found, it should be related to the spatial discretisation of the fluid.

If the average triangulation edge length is much shorter than the lattice unit as depicted in Figure 5.9 (c), the interpolated fluid velocity at these two

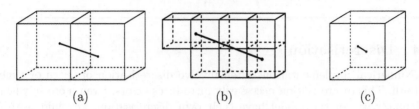

FIGURE 5.9: Triangulation edge length vs. discretisation of the fluid. (a) Edge length is comparable to the lattice grid size. (b) The edge spans over several lattice units. (c) The edge is much smaller than the lattice grid size.

nodes is very similar, they tend to move together but they influence the fluid (by applying force to lattice nodes) much further than the radius of the local elastic deformations that they feel.

If the triangulation edge length is significantly longer than the lattice unit, Figure 5.9 (b), there are lattice nodes close to the membrane that should feel the effect of the membrane, but they do not, since there is no triangulation node in any of the cubes to which they belong. This is not correct, since this means locally inconsistent behavior of the fluid close to the membrane.

Therefore, a reasonable compromise is to have average mesh edge length approximately equal to the fluid lattice resolution as in Figure 5.9 (a). A good rule of thumb is that if a triangulation edge passes through the lattice cube, the eight lattice nodes belonging to this cube should interact with one mesh node of this triangulation edge. Of course, this does not mean that we should not use triangulations where, for example, one triangular face lies inside the cube, this is meant more as an order of magnitude approximation.

5.4.2   Fluid boundary discretisation

When considering the spatial resolution of the fluid lattice, it is important to keep in mind, what kind of boundary conditions are used. The simplest case is to use the periodic boundary conditions, i.e. no walls. This may be useful for simulations of large domains where we can take advantage of the periodicity to decrease the computational time (see also Section 5.2) and as a by-product to avoid treatment of the boundaries.

However, more often than not, the desired applications do require some boundaries - either as actual boundaries of simulated chambers or as obstacles in periodically repeating blocks that have periodic boundary conditions. And so it becomes necessary to consider what should happen at the boundaries.

Usually, one imposes no-slip boundary conditions, i.e. Cauchy boundary conditions with fluid velocity at the boundary set to zero. This corresponds

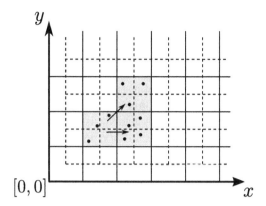

FIGURE 5.10: Shift of a fluid lattice (dashed grid) with respect to the origin in a two-dimensional case.

to typical situations with microfluidic chambers and the physical intuition we might have from observing the flow of the river at the river bank.

Fluid boundaries

There are several types of the fluid boundaries. We have extensively discussed the fluid-object boundary and the no-slip condition on the moving membrane surface in Section 3.5.2.

Then there are the boundaries, which are walls and obstacles, as introduced in Chapter 2 and discussed from a practical point of view in this section. These are non-deformable stationary boundaries present in microfluidic devices.

Finally, in case of biological and computational flows in the vascular system, one has to consider a combination of the previous types. The walls of veins are practically stationary, however, they are elastic. This results in a different type of cell-wall interaction, which is not considered in this book.

An alternative is to impose non-zero velocity at the boundaries. This can be useful for examining the cell behavior in shear flow, such as described in Section 4.3.2. To achieve both of these in LBM, a bounce-back condition is often used [196], which assumes walls located halfway between the lattice nodes.

While we do not discuss the details of the LBM method here, we need to mention some issues arising from discretisation of fluid near boundaries, since they might influence the cell simulations. Consider a channel with dimensions $20 \times 10 \times 10$ with a wall of thickness 1 at the bottom and on the top.

The idea of dividing the space into little cubes also helps in understanding why in practice the lattice for the fluid is often shifted by [0.5, 0.5, 0.5] with respect to the origin. The LB nodes thus correspond to the center of these little cubes, as depicted in Figure 5.10 and the fluid lattice node with indices [1, 2, 3] has physical coordinates [1.5, 2.5, 3.5].

Next consider a cylindrical obstacle, centered at given location, e.g. [5, 5, 5], having a defined radius, e.g. $r = 2$. A 2D slice of this situation is shown in Figure 5.11. All fluid nodes inside the column (thick crosses) are treated as boundary nodes and thus the fluid velocity here is zero. The thin crosses denote some other points where the velocity is zero; these are the points inside the cubes, whose all vertices are boundary points (thick crosses).

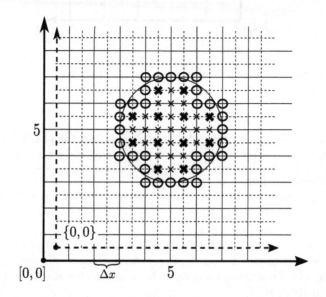

FIGURE 5.11: The desired boundary is a cylinder centered at [5, 5] with radius $r = 2$. For simplicity, we provide an example which is a 2D slice of a 3D situation. All lattice nodes (intersections of dashed lines, with origin at [0, 0]) located inside the circle (thick crosses) are boundary nodes and fluid velocity in them is zero. Fluid velocity is also zero inside the lattice cubes defined by the boundary nodes (thin crosses). Fluid velocity is non-zero in all lattice cubes, where at least one vertex has non-zero velocity (circles). In this figure we also see that the fluid nodes indices (intersections of dashed lines) are shifted by $\Delta x/2$ relative to physical coordinates (full lines, with origin at [0, 0]). This is due to the bounce-back boundary condition that is used for LBM.

Now look at the physical position [4, 4]. It is clearly inside the obstacle, because $(4 - 5)^2 + (4 - 5)^2 < r^2$. And it has non-zero velocity because $v_{[4,4]}$ is interpolated from neighboring lattice nodes, one of which (the one with index=[3,3] physical coordinates [3.5, 3.5]) has non-zero velocity. This means that instead of a cylindrical column, we effectively have a cross-like structure as an obstacle.

This effect is less pronounced when the ratio of column radius to lattice spacing is larger but what it signifies is that our linear interpolation scheme (tri-linear in fact, since we are in three dimensions) makes the method only first-order accurate, and with cylindrical obstacles we do not have no-slip on the boundary.

5.4.3 Creating triangulations of objects

Once we have an analytic expression for a surface, such as (3.1) there are a number of softwares that can be used to triangulate it, e.g. Gmsh [74] or Salome [165]. The goal is to get as regular triangulation as possible. By regular we mean that the triangles are close to equilateral and they all have approximately the same size. Consequently, most vertices should have six neighbors.

Things to ponder

Is it possible to get a triangulation of sphere (or RBC) such that all triangles are equilateral?

Is it possible to get a triangulation of sphere (or RBC) such that all vertices have exactly six neighbors?

Rings in triangulation

An easy way to triangulate an RBC surface in Gmsh is as follows. Consider one octant in Cartesian coordinates. Create a quarter circle in the xy-plane. Define the RBC curve in the xz and yz planes. Gmsh can now triangulate the surface in 3D bounded by these three curves. To get the whole RBC mesh, rotate this surface three times by 90 degrees to get the three other octants and join the four of them together. Finally, mirror everything with negative z coordinates and join.

While this approach using rotational and mirror symmetry is fast and straightforward, it is not ideal. The resulting triangulation has an *equatorial ring* and two perpendicular *meridian rings*, Figure 5.12. These become prominent in certain situations, e.g. when simulating the optical tweezers stretching experiment from Section 4.3.1, which is undesirable. Clearly, we do not want discretisation or numerical artefacts such as this one to influence the results of validation experiments.

There is not much we can do about removing the rings in the first place, because we need to specify the surface somehow, but there are a few other things that can be done.

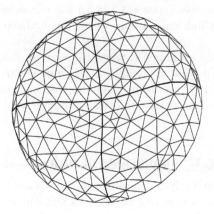

FIGURE 5.12: Meridian rings as artefacts of rotational symmetry when generating the mesh of RBC.

Using noise to get rid of rings

One possible way to get rid of the rings is to slightly move all the triangulation points. This is easier for spheres than for RBCs, because for spheres this simply means generating three small random numbers that represent rotations around the three Cartesian axes. Then we can randomly rotate each point independently, project it back onto the sphere surface and keep the triangle incidences. The drawbacks of this approach are that it is problematic for surfaces other than spheres and that we are willingly decreasing the regularity of the mesh.

Things to ponder
What other approaches could be used to introduce noise?

Incorrect use of projections for triangulations

What if instead of removing the rings, we could avoid them in the first place? Maybe we have a regular triangulation of a sphere that we would like to use for creation of RBC triangulation. We take all the points except the *equatorial* points with $z = 0$ and project them onto the RBC curve (3.1) by changing their z-coordinates accordingly. When all is said and done, we have a triangulation of RBC, but not a very regular one. The areas with higher curvature (towards the rim) will have more points and less regular triangles, while the two dimples in the center will have fewer points.

Similarly, it is not desirable to use stretching of spheres to get triangulations of ellipsoids, etc.

Triangulations by successive refinement and outward projection

All of the approaches presented so far had significant drawbacks. So how does one actually create a good triangulation? We can start with a regular icosahedron - a solid which has 20 triangular faces. It has 12 vertices, each of which has 5 neighbors. Each of the triangular faces can be replaced by 4 new smaller triangles by dividing each edge in half and connecting the new points. These new points are then projected outward on the enclosing sphere surface and the whole process, illustrated in Figure 5.13, is repeated. The result is a very regular triangulation - all points but the 12 initial vertices have 6 neighbors.

The only minor drawback is that the number of vertices increases geometrically in each step and we cannot create a mesh with an arbitrary number of points.

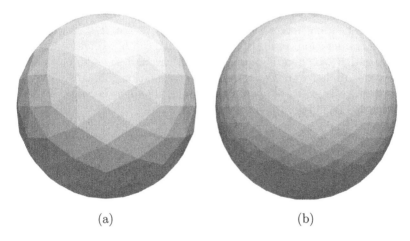

(a)   (b)

FIGURE 5.13: Mesh refinement. (a) Coarse mesh with 122 nodes. (b) Mesh with 482 nodes obtained from the coarse mesh by splitting each triangle into four new triangles and projecting new vertices onto the circumscribed sphere.

RBC triangulation from a sphere by decreasing volume

Using a regular triangulation of a sphere, a similarly regular triangulation of RBC might be produced by decreasing the volume of the sphere with RBC surface down to the volume of RBC. A shape very similar to (3.1) emerges thanks to elastic energy minimizing principles.

5.5 Computational complexity and parallelisation

The analysis of computational complexity is essentially done to answer the question of the computational time and computer memory that are needed to simulate a model of the given size and detail. With the current state of computational resources in general and the simplicity of the presented models in particular, we face a problem of computational time and not the problem of not enough memory. Therefore in the following, we make a rough estimate of the number of operations needed to perform a simulation of a given size. We use the *O-notation* that has been established for characterisation of computational complexity, which gives the terms to the largest order.

Think about one cell with n mesh nodes and t mesh triangles. How many interactions are evaluated at each time step?

- There are $3t/2$ stretching interactions, because each triangle has three edges, each of which is counted twice, since it belongs to two neighboring triangles. Each of these interactions needs $O(1)$ operations. The situation with bending interactions is similar, there are $3t/2$ of them and with $O(1)$ operations each. However, we have combined all local interactions together, so there is no second loop through the edges. While there is some duplicity (*triplicity* in fact) in calculation of local area forces - each triangle is evaluated each time any of its edges is considered, this still means $O(1)$ operations with respect to t.

- Similarly, both global surface and global volume conservation interactions are evaluated together. First there is a loop over the triangles that calculates the current global surface and global volume. And then there is a second loop over the triangles to apply the forces. In total, there are $O(1)$ operations these $2t$ times.

Thus, one cell requires $O(t)$ operations every time step. In a simulation with N cells, we have

- $O(Nt)$ operations for the elasticity of cells.

- Cell-cell interactions: Since we have a particle-based model and cell-cell interactions are evaluated on a particle-particle basis (see Section 3.6), the first calculation would give $(nN)^2/2$ interactions, each with $O(1)$ operations. In practice, the particles that are too far do not need to interact. How do we learn they are too far? We could calculate their distance, but this is not a way to go because that would still leave us with $(nN)^2/2$ distance calculations. So what do we do instead?

We keep a Verlet list of particles as depicted in Figure 5.14. Only particles that are on this list enter the distance calculation (for non-bonded

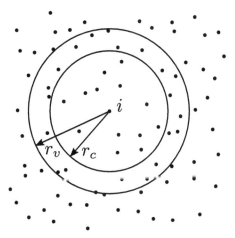

FIGURE 5.14: Verlet list [69]: a particle i interacts only with particles within the radious r_c and keeps a list of particles within the sphere with radius $r_v > r_c$.

interactions) and only those that have the distance smaller than the cut-off radius actually interact ($O(nN)$ calculations). Once in a while, when any particle moves more than $r_v - r_c$, all the distances are recomputed and the Verlet lists updated ($O((nN)^2)$ calculations). This is all nice and good, but now comes the part where the seasoned computational scientists roll their eyes and normal people tear their hair out. How do we choose the value r_v, which essentially determines how many particles make the list?

Obviously, we do not want it too small: while it would limit the number of particles on the list (fewer distance calculations) it would also mean more frequent update of the list (more distance calculations). We do not want it too large either: such a setup would mean that we do not update the Verlet lists very often (fewer distance calculations), but also there are more particles on the list and thus more need to be checked for interactions (more distance calculations). There is an optimum value somewhere between these two extremes, but it is not at all obvious what it is.

Specifically in ESPResSo, this can be tuned using the parameter *skin*. Essentially, for a given simulation setup, a few values are tried for a short time and the resulting computational times are compared. Not too scientific? Well, sometimes the selection of simulation parameters is more of a magic than science and those who have not acquired the magical powers through experience have to rely on the brute force calculations. To summarise, no matter what value the parameter *skin* has (and the only restriction is that it has to be strictly less than half the spatial step Δx), the results of the simulation are the same, even though the time to achieve them may vary dramatically.

- Particle movement: This depends on the particular integration of Newton's equation of motion. It is possible to make the number of operations linear with respect to the number of particles and linear with respect to time discretisation.

- Lattice-Boltzmann calculations: This depends on the particular implementation of the LBM (in ESPResSo this is a multi-relaxation scheme), but in general the number of operations is linear with respect to the number of spatial discretisation nodes. In terms of memory, it is necessary to save the population information in all lattice-Boltzmann nodes (thus $n_x \times n_y \times n_z \times 19$ array for D3Q19 scheme) and keep additional space of the same size for the newly calculated values. It is possible to perform both the streaming and collision steps at the same time, so that each node has to be read and written only once.

- Cell-wall interactions: This is similar to cell-cell interactions and should be $(Nnn_b)^2/2$, where n_b is the number of boundaries.

Overall, we see that the bottleneck arises from cell-cell interactions, if they are not treated carefully.

Parallelisation

Dry silicon has a great advantage over the wet carbon. We can perform calculations and computations that have not been possible just recently. We can perform simulation studies such as the one described in Section 6.4, and if the computational domain is too large, we have the luxury to parallelise - split it into smaller pieces, each of which is computed separately.

Going back to the silicone-carbon comparison, where the carbon-based units automatically take care of many processes that run in parallel (such as, we can breathe, beat our hearts, wave with our hands and talk simultaneously without the need to micromanage everything), the silicone-based units have to be told exactly what, when and how to compute. And if they are supposed to compute in parallel they need to communicate with each other.

What do they talk about? Think for example about the cell-cell interactions. The whole computational domain is divided into a few parts. Cells which are somewhere in the centers of these parts, also have their neighbors in the same parts. Cell-cell interactions can be evaluated without any issues. But what about cells at the border of the subdomain? Some of their neighbors are available, but some are already in the next subdomain. To calculate their interactions, the subdomains have to have the information about the cells close to the boundary of the neighboring regions. So this is the topic of

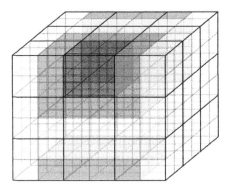

FIGURE 5.15: The simulation box is divided into 27 local boxes, each containing eight computational cells. The local boxes are lined with thicker black lines, computational cells with thinner black lines. One local box is highlighted in dark grey and the corresponding communication region is shown in light grey.

conversation. And the same holds for the fluid, which in case of the fairly local lattice-Boltzmann method, fortunately does not make for a very extensive communication.

Here we examine these ideas in some more detail, however for particulars of a massive parallelisation of RBC simulations we refer the reader to, e.g. [33]. As depicted in Figure 5.15, the simulation box can be divided into several local boxes. Each of the local boxes is then divided into computational cells. The size of the computational cell has to be as small as possible, but at the same time has to be larger than the longest bonded interaction. In our case this means that a biological cell has to fit into it, since the global surface and volume interactions span the whole cell. The computational cells at the edges of the local box form the *halo region*. Information from this region is communicated to the neighboring local box.

In case of periodic boundary conditions (such as those depicted in Figure 5.15), it is possible that the halo region is located on the opposite side of the simulation box.

While the minimal size of the computational cells has a strict restriction, the local boxes can be determined by the user as long as their dimensions divide the dimensions of the whole simulation box and are multiples of the spatial discretisation step. The dimensions of the computational cells then have to divide the dimensions of the local box.

In the following, we show an example setup that can be used for parallel computations. Suppose we want to simulate a chamber with dimensions

$120 \times 48 \times 48$ (in non-dimensionalised settings) and some red blood cells. The diameter of RBC is about 8 and if we consider possible stretching, we can assume that the longest range for bonded interaction will be 12. The cutoff radius for non-bonded interactions, i.e. membrane collision and soft-sphere interaction with walls, is much smaller - up to 0.5. So the minimal size of the computational cells should be 12 (actually $12 + skin$. We discussed *skin* in more detail in Section 5.5 within a bullet list concerning cell-cell interactions. For the purposes of this explanation, we can neglect it).

In ESPResSo, we could use the system's global variable `min_global_cut` set to 12, which would guarantee that every computational cell would be of dimension at least $12 \times 12 \times 12$. Thus, every computational core (one local box) will see the particles far enough to include the whole blood cell. To reiterate, all particles, bonds, boundaries, etc., need to be specified before setting `min_global_cut`, because this variable triggers calculation of dimensions of local boxes and if any long-range items were added later, they would compromise the division into subdomains.

If we have eight nodes available, the simulation box will thus be divided into eight local boxes, probably each having dimensions $60 \times 24 \times 24$. In this case, the computational cell would have dimensions $12 \times 12 \times 12$, but if the whole domain was $120 \times 40 \times 40$ and local boxes $60 \times 20 \times 20$, the computational cell would have forced dimensions $12 \times 20 \times 20$. The command to then run the script in parallel is

```
mpirun -np 8 ./pypresso script.py
```

The `mpirun` refers to MPI (Message Passing Interface) that needs to be enabled, for example by installing OpenMpi [71], and then compiling ESPResSo with MPI. np denotes the number of processors.

Similarly, if we had 16 nodes available, we would run

```
mpirun -np 16 ./pypresso script.py
```

With `min_global_cut` set to 12 we would probably have 16 local boxes with dimensions $30 \times 24 \times 24$ each and computational cells with dimensions $15 \times 12 \times 12$ each.

Chapter 6

Applications

6.1 Microfluidic cell manipulation

Blood and its flow have been of interest to biomedical professionals for a long time since it is a fluid crucial to life. The second half of the last century saw experiments at cell scale, probing various cell properties and development of applications that involved cell handling or manipulation. But it was in the last two decades that we have seen a major development and applications branching out in various directions, such as the following:

- Lab-on-a-chip (LOC) - The idea is to miniaturise a laboratory to a portable chip that uses only small amounts of fluid. This area even has its own journal (appropriately titled Lab-on-a-chip) and encompasses several of the following more specific points.

- Point-of-care (POC) diagnostics - This concept is related to the previous point, since such devices often include LOC. For a review of several

POC microfluidic devices and especially the issues related to their development and deployment for use, see [29].

- Lateral flow tests - These are one specific example of POC diagnostics. Typically they use a membrane or paper strip to indicate the presence of markers such as pathogen antigens or host antibodies. On the paper or on the membrane, the (blood) sample induces capillary action without user intervention. As the sample flows, it combines with the labeling reagents embedded in the paper or membrane and flows over an area that contains capture molecules. The results are then interpreted when the person looks at visible band(s) on the test. These kinds of tests are used for pregnancy, infections, etc.

- Blood glucose test - One of the best known tests that analyses a drop of blood taken from a finger.

- Mixing - Mixing is needed in several applications such as blood typing or agglutination-based assays. It is a non-trivial problem since if there is a pressure difference between the two liquids that should be merged together, a surge backflow may happen [199].

- Sorting/separation of cells - Sorting and separation may be based on several different ideas. In continuous flow, individual components may be deflected from the main direction of flow by means of a force field (electric, magnetic, acoustic, optical, etc.) or by clever positioning of obstacles in combination with laminar flow profiles. Some of the reported methods are miniaturised versions of larger scale methods, while others are only possible in microfluidic regimes [146].

- Drug delivery - Various techniques can work at various scales. At the cellular level, the most widely investigated principle is the concentration gradient generator integrated with a cell culture platform that is responsible for the drug delivery. At the tissue level, the focus is on smart particles, which carry the drugs to the desired locations. And at the organism level, micro-needles and implantable devices capable of handling fluid can be used to deliver the drugs [140].

- Separation of viruses from blood - Devices capable of such task may contain micro-patterned arrays of macro-porous materials and perform size-exclusion [182].

With the rapid development in this area, it is peculiar though, why many of these concepts remain in the academic proof-of-concept studies, some of which have been around for more than 10 years now. We do not see very many of them in everyday practice, even when accounting for the long delay involved in translating medical research to practical use. Yes, the blood glucose test and a few others are available, but it is not yet standard to encounter microfluidic assisted diagnostics or treatment when visiting a doctor or hospital these days. That makes us wonder about the possible issues.

The first one that comes to mind is money. Maybe there are the usual problems with investment or theoretical development focused more on innovation and not so much on a specific product? While the former may be present, the amount of money present in the pharmaceutical industry suggests that robust techniques with practical potential should be able to find financial support.

Another issue could be the technology itself. Microfluidic devices rely on glass, silicone or PDMS, which probably are not the most suitable materials for mass production. If this is the case, more research is needed to transfer the knowledge into paper based or (biodegradable) plastic devices that would be more suitable.

And then there is of course the integration. A microfluidic device has to integrate several steps between obtaining the sample and giving the result to the patient. If any of them is faulty, it capsizes the whole concept even if the rest of them are fine.

Finally, the longer a major breakthrough takes, the worse sentiment it has to overcome. If a lot of money has been invested with not too much to show for it, then the general scepticism might be that maybe it is not worth it.

One thing is clear though. Due to the very nature of the problems, in the design phase, the microfluidic applications may benefit from simulations a lot. And therefore, in this chapter, we show a few applications where a model such as the one described in previous chapters can be used. We start with periodic obstacle arrays where we first look at possibilities of estimating cell capture rates and then on ways to use deterministic lateral displacement for maximizing the capture rate.

The next section looks at the larger scale - design of blood pumps and other ventricular assisting devices and how modeling the stress on single cells can assist in such design.

Single-cell stress can also be estimated and we discuss the cell damage index and computational estimation of hemolysis.

The final section in this chapter showcases an investigation of wall roughness and its impact of cell flow in microfluidic device.

6.2   Designing a simulation study

What all the following applications have in common is the fact that they have a quantity that can be used to compare different devices. Therefore we can perform a simulation study and examine the effect of the device and flow parameters on this quantity. Here we summarise a few points that we take into account when designing a simulation study.

- **Parameter ranges** The main advantage of simulation study is the ability to perform a multitude of experiments under various conditions. One needs to think in advance what the variables are and in what ranges do their values vary. These ranges should then be reasonably sampled and simulations should be run for suitable combinations of parameter values.

- **Comparability of simulation runs** There will certainly also be values that need to be kept constant across all simulations. This might be straightforward, e.g. dimensions of the simulation box, or quite tricky, c.g. fixed flow rate if the total volume of the box changes due to obstacles. In any case, it is a good practice to think what are the *constants* in the simulation setup and verify that they indeed do not vary.

- **Initial conditions and randomness** If your simulation study includes a stochastic aspect, i.e. anything that is random, this implies that it is not sufficient to run any individual setup once and take the results. The simulation should be repeated several times and the observables should be averaged. Confidence intervals may be used to infer the number of necessary replications. The randomness most often occurs with respect to initial conditions, such as in seeding of cells.

- **Observed quantities** When designing a simulation study, we know what we want to measure, but it is a good idea to observe, i.e. also measure other quantities, and even those whose values we *know*. This serves for confirmation that our system is set up right. Ideally, we should think about some conserved quantities (cell volumes, energy of the system, etc.) that can also be monitored as a basic sanity check that everything is working as it is supposed to.

- **Interpretation of results** When looking at the results we got and any implications they might lead to, we have to consider the assumptions made beforehand. Are they still valid for our implications? If something is truly unexpected, before accepting it, we need to go back to the design of the simulation study and try to verify the steps that lead to our discovery.

6.3   Periodic obstacle arrays (POAs)

Periodic obstacle arrays are parts of microfluidic devices where the flow chamber contains many (at the order of hundreds or thousands) obstacles of various shapes and sizes whose purpose is to maximize the cell-obstacle contact opportunities or direct the flow in a desired way. From a simulation perspective, these are rather nice, because the periodicity allows investigation over smaller domains instead of the whole large device, Figure 6.1. For more details, we refer the reader to Section 5.2.

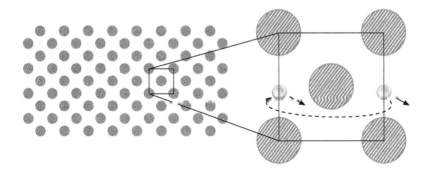

FIGURE 6.1: A periodic obstacle array - view from top.

Usually, and also in the following two simulation studies, the obstacles are cylindrical, however other types, such as square [191], triangular [168], etc. have been investigated.

Periodic obstacle arrays are often used for the separation of cells. If the array is designed in such a way that consecutive rows of obstacles are shifted by a small offset with respect to the previous rows, as depicted in Figure 6.2, smaller particles or smaller cells will follow a zig-zag trajectory, while larger particles or cells will always be bounced up [128]. At the end of the device, the cells may be collected in two outputs, now separated according to their size.

A similar idea may be used to separate cells of the same size according to their deformability. A deformable cell elongates when passing the obstacle and thus remains in a region leading to a zig-zag trajectory. A non-deformable cell protrudes to the bounce-up region and is bounced up to the next row of obstacles. This idea has been analysed in [108] with promising results.

Another known biomedical application of periodic obstacle arrays is the capture of rare cells [137, 179]. A specific kind of rare cell that is often considered is the circulating tumor cell that leaves the primary cancer tumor, enters the bloodstream and is linked with the onset of metastases. Analysis of blood samples of cancer patients can reveal the amount of such cells in blood and be used for diagnostics or monitoring of response to treatment. The analysis relies on capturing the rare cells from the sample using a microfluidic device. capture!of rare cells The biological background of rare cell capture is based on functionalisation of the obstacle surface by proteins (ligands) that can bind other proteins (receptors) that are expressed on the cell surface. When a cell touches a functionalised wall, ligands may bind to receptors creating bonds.

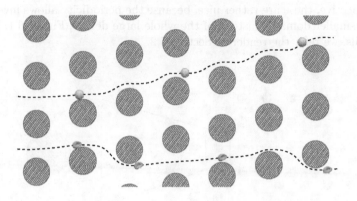

FIGURE 6.2: Size-based separation of cells.

If a sufficient number of bonds are created, cells may adhere to the function-alised surface. Quantification of the efficiency of such rare cell capture may be tricky. One can model the capture directly by introducing the formation of bonds. This is however difficult from implementation as well as the calibration side. We talk about this approach in Section 7.2.

Another approach is to lump the effect of the individual bonds and create a model of capture rate with lumped parameters. The model takes into account variables such as size of the cell-obstacle contact or duration of the contact. These variables determine the likelihood of cells attachment, when the cell-obstacle contact has specific size and duration. This approach is discussed in more detail in Section 6.4.

We can even go further and again lump the effect of the cell-obstacle size and duration and simply count the number of such contacts during the passage of the cell through the device. Considering the large number of obstacles that the cell may pass by, we can simply evaluate the collision rate as a fraction of actual hits to total possible hits. The higher this fraction (thus the higher the collision rate), the higher is the probability that during such a collision, the cell would actually adhere to the obstacle and be captured. This approach of capture quantification is discussed in Section 6.5.

6.4   Capture rates for rare cells in POAs

During the optimisation of microfluidic device design, such as in [175], many simplifying assumptions are made, e.g. the model uses only tracers instead of actual cells or one-way interaction of fluid and the cells immersed in it is used instead of full two-way interaction. However, there is no such thing as free lunch. When we aim to have spatial resolution that captures the cell deformations and include full fluid-cell and cell-cell interactions, the trade-off has to show up somewhere else. It does in terms of spatial domain: we simulate one periodic block instead of the whole device. And it also shows up in terms of temporal domain: we simulate one or few cell passes of this periodic block with various initial conditions and then use data post-processing to evaluate the capture rates over many passes.

6.4.1 Models for calculating capture rates

Experiments using a Hele-Shaw chamber with functionalised surface were used to determine the dependence of capture rate of human prostate cancer cells on shear stress near the wall [166]. The modeling of individual bonds formation between cells and functionalised surfaces requires inclusion of parameters whose physical values are largely unavailable. To circumvent this, reduced models can be used. In [43], the authors present a relatively simple exponential model for cell capture in linear shear flow. This model predicts the capture rate of adhesion in a simple channel as

$$P_a \simeq m_r m_l K_a^0 A_c \, \exp\left[-\frac{\lambda F}{k_B T}\right], \tag{6.1}$$

where m_r, m_l is the surface density of receptors and ligands, K_a^0 is the association constant at zero load of the ligand-receptor pair, A_c is the area of interaction between the cell and functionalised surface, F is magnitude of force per unit ligand-receptor pair, λ is a characteristic length of the ligand-receptor bond and $k_B T$ is the Boltzmann thermal energy.

The quantity F is difficult to determine and is often approximated using the dislodging hydrodynamic force of the cell moving under a given shear stress. Assuming uniform distribution of the dislodging force over all active bond-ligand couples, the force F per unit ligand-receptor bond can be expressed as the ratio between the total dislodging force F_{dis} and the area of interaction A_c multiplied by the surface density of the receptors m_r, that is

$$F = \frac{F_{dis}}{m_r A_c}. \tag{6.2}$$

Combining (6.1) with (6.2), the capture rate can be expressed as

$$P_a \simeq m_r m_l K_a^0 A_c \, \exp\left[-\frac{\lambda}{k_B T}\frac{F_{dis}}{m_r A_c}\right]. \tag{6.3}$$

In linear shear flow, the dislodging force F_{dis} can be linearised near the wall and thus F_{dis} is taken proportional to the shear stress τ. In [175], the authors suggested to group multiple parameters into two lumped parameters A and B resulting in the following capture model:

$$P_a \simeq A \, \exp\left[-B\tau\right]. \tag{6.4}$$

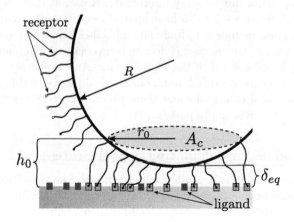

FIGURE 6.3: Spherical cell adhered to a surface, redrawn from [43].

The parameters A and B were calibrated using experimental data and simulations of the microfluidic device with periodically repeating blocks of cylindrical obstacles. Assuming the same cell and surface chemistry, the parameters m_r, m_l, K_a^0, λ, k_B and T in (6.3) are constant and they may be safely included under lumped parameters A and B. However, the area of interaction between cell and device surface, A_c, varies with different τ. In fact, cells may deform under the shear stress and may have ellipsoidal shapes with different aspect ratios for different shear stresses. In [43], the authors analyse ellipsoidal particles and they show that A_c changes under different aspect ratios. The contact area also varies with parameters of obstacles, e.g. increases with increasing column radius.

Another reason to keep A_c variable in the capture model is that such a model would also be usable in dense suspensions, where the cell contact area may vary due to cell-cell collisions.

These considerations have led to the proposal of the following model for cell capture [22]:

$$P_a \simeq aA_c \, \exp\left[-b\frac{\tau}{A_c}\right]. \tag{6.5}$$

Similarly as in [175], several parameters are grouped, however A_c is kept variable. To calibrate the new model parameters a and b, the contact area A_c^* for the experiment in [166] is computed as follows. The cells used in experiments are considered spherical with radius $R = 17.5/2 = 8.75\mu m$. The contact area A_c is defined as projection of that part of the cell that is in the distance at most h_0 from the surface. Moreover, the distance of the cell from the surface during the adhesion contact is at least δ_{eq}, see Figure 6.3. A physiologically relevant value for $\delta_{eq} = 5 \times 10^{-9}m$ is taken from [43]. h_0 is the length of the combined receptor-ligand couple. However, there are different values reported in different sources. In the pioneering work [87], the ratio of bond length to cell radius is reported in the range from 0.002 to 0.01. The work [106] reports $h_0 = 5 \times 10^{-8}m$ and [58] reports $h_0 = 3.5 \times 10^{-7}m$. The following computation uses the value $h_0 = 5 \times 10^{-8}m$. Using the radius $R = 8.75 \times 10^{-6}m$, we can compute $A_c^* = \pi r_0^2$, where r_0 satisfies

$$
\begin{aligned}
r_0^2 + (R - (h_0 - \delta_{eq}))^2 &= R^2 \\
r_0^2 &= 2R(h_0 - \delta_{eq}) - (h_0 - \delta_{eq})^2 \\
r_0^2 &= 17.5(0.05 - 0.005) - (0.05 - 0.005)^2 \\
r_0^2 &\doteq 0.785\mu m^2,
\end{aligned}
$$

which results in $A_c^* \doteq 2.47\mu m^2$ and subsequently in

$$
\begin{aligned}
a &= A/A_c^* = 0.0344/2.47 = 13.927 \times 10^{-3}s^{-1}\mu m^{-2} \\
b &= BA_c^* = 85.5 \times 2.47 = 211.185Pa^{-1}\mu m^2. \quad (6.6)
\end{aligned}
$$

Note, the P_a in (6.5) is not a probability that the cell will be captured in the corresponding pass through the device, but rather a characteristic measure that can be used to compare different device designs.

In the simulation, the contact area is determined as follows:

```
# calculation of contact area
npoints_in_contact = 0
for point in rbc.mesh.points:
    if vec_distance(point.get_pos(),cyl_center) < threshold:
        npoints_in_contact += 1
contact_area = (npoints_in_contact / cell.mesh.get_n_nodes()) * \
cell.volume()
```

and the capture rate is calculated as

```
# calculation of capture rate
shear_stress = fluid_viscosity * fluid_density * cell_velocity_projection \
/ cell_dist_to_obstacle
if contact_area > 0:
    capture_rate_for_obstacle = (A/Ac)*contact_area*exp(-(B*Ac) * \
    shear_stress/contact_area)
else:
    capture_rate_for_obstacle = 0
```

6.4.2 Performing a simulation study

Here we look at one periodic block of the array, Figure 6.4, which was a rectangular box with five cylindrical obstacles or their parts. The parameters of interest were the radius of obstacle and volume fraction of red blood cells.

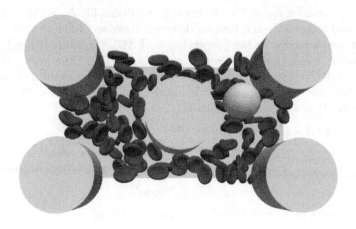

FIGURE 6.4: One block of a periodic obstacle array.

The increase in radius leads to several effects: Assuming constant volumetric flow rate, the shear stress at the obstacle boundaries gets higher and so decreases the capture rate. The area of the cell-obstacle contact may get larger at higher shear stresses, because the cells deform more. This affects the capture rate in the opposite way, i.e. makes it increase. Finally, the duration of cell-obstacle contact may get longer, which again causes an increase in capture rate. Simulations can show details about such interplay.

6.4.3   Parameter ranges

We have already identified the two variables to examine: column radius and volume fraction of red blood cells. The dimensions of the periodic block to be simulated were $100 \times 50 \times 30 \mu m^3$. This meant there were five columns (four of them partial) in this domain. For the column radius, we have considered the range 7-13μm. The lower number corresponds to a small but already noticeable obstacle (with respect to the red blood cells). The upper bound corresponds to the largest columns that still leave some space between them for a rare cell to pass at different locations. We have sampled this parameter space uniformly - performing simulations with radii 7, 9, 11, 13μm.

For volume fraction, we were limited by computational times. The initial idea was to look at three different volume fractions, e.g. 3%, 6% and 9%, however, since the free volume of the simulated chamber changes with radius of obstacles and the volume fractions would not be exact across different simulations, we simply kept the number of cells constant (10, 50, 100) and kept track of the actual volume fraction, Table 6.1.

	$n_{cell} = 10$	$n_{cell} = 50$	$n_{cell} = 100$
$r = 7$	2.79	5.42	8.71
$r = 9$	2.92	5.67	9.10
$r = 11$	3.09	6.00	9.64
$r = 13$	3.33	6.46	10.38

TABLE 6.1: Hematocrit values (in %) for different cell counts. The values were computed as volume occupied by all cells (RBCs and rare cell) divided by total free volume inside the chamber. Radii in μm. Values from [22].

6.4.4 Comparability of simulation runs - Fixed flow rate

The free volume inside our chamber varies with variable column radius, but we would nevertheless like to keep the flow rate fixed. Experimentally measured maximum flow rate in microfluidic devices varies from around 0.007-0.008m/s in [19] to 0.017-0.018m/s in [50]. The devices that use antibody coated surfaces typically need slow flow so that the cells come into contact with obstacles and have time to form the adhesion bonds.

Therefore in our simulations, we have kept the maximum velocity at the lower end of this range: between 0.005 and 0.008m/s. The volumetric flow rate Q is calculated as an integral of velocity profile at the $x = 0$ plane. We have kept the volumetric flow rate constant at $Q = 2.775 \times 10^{-12} m^3/s \doteq 10^{-2} ml/h$ (this is for the one periodic block, thus only a fraction of the total volumetric flow rate through the device).

The fluid was initialised using an external force that resulted in the desired volumetric flow rate and it has typically reached steady state by the time the rare cell has traveled 2-3% of the total trajectory. We have simulated one pass of the rare cell through the chamber. Later we include details on a comparison of our results calculated from these simulations to results from long simulation that allow the rare cell to make several passes of the chamber.

The rare cells were modeled as spheres with radius $r_{rare} = 8.75\mu m$ using a triangular mesh with 727 nodes. RBCs have a typical biconcave shape with diameter $r_{RBC} = 3.91\mu m$, and we have used a triangular mesh with 141 nodes.

6.4.5 Initial conditions and randomness

For each combination of column radius (four values) and each number of cells (10, 50, 100) we have used 10 different seedings of rare cell on the left-hand side of the simulated chamber ($x = 1$). The 10 different seedings of rare cell were regularly spaced in the opening between the two columns. We have repeated each of these simulations 10 times with different (random) RBC seedings. This resulted in the total number of 1200 performed simulations.

6.4.6   Observed characteristics

First let us look at the expected: The distribution of red blood cells at the right-hand side of the chamber ($x = 100$) after one pass has a characteristic two-peak shape, Figure 6.5, which is due to fluid streamlines that, in general, take the cells away from the central point between the columns due to the central obstacle. Note, that in these and also subsequent figures, the axes do not have the same scale.

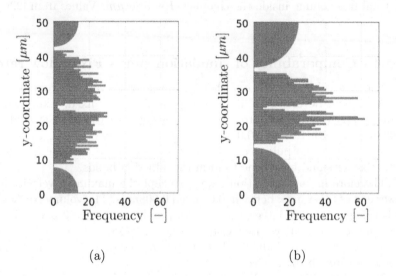

(a)   (b)

FIGURE 6.5: Distribution of y-coordinates of RBCs between two columns: (a) $r = 7\mu m$, (b) $r = 13\mu m$.

Also as expected, the rare cell trajectories behave differently in simulations with a small number of RBCs and a large number of RBCs, Figure 6.6. While in simulations with 10 RBCs, where they basically do not come into contact with other cells, they fall into the same pattern, in simulations with 100 RBCs this pattern is quite often disturbed due to cell-cell contacts.

Now for the capture rates we set out to observe: In our investigation, we assume the obstacle density $400mm^{-2}$, since we have two obstacles per $50 \times 100\mu m^2$. This roughly corresponds to the microfluidic device described in [137], which had 78,000 (significantly larger) microposts covering the area of $970mm^2$. It also means about 20 passes of the periodic chamber per mm. Thus for a specific microfluidic device with length L, the total number of passes of a periodic block for a rare cell would be calculated as $N_{pass} \approx L \times 20$. For our capture rate calculations, we have used $N_{pass} = 400$.

We would like to determine the typical distribution of the y-coordinate of rare cell at the right end of the simulation chamber and use it in the calculation of the capture rate over N_{pass} passes of the chamber without the

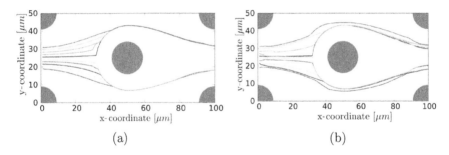

FIGURE 6.6: Typical rare cell trajectories. Each line corresponds to a rare cell center in different rare cell seeding: (a) simulations with 10 RBCs, (b) simulations with 100 RBCs.

need to actually simulate such a long process. Clearly, the rare cell positions will not be distributed uniformly between the two cylindrical obstacles. To determine the typical distribution of y-coordinate of a rare cell we start with uniform distribution.

With a fixed cell count we use the simulations with 10 regularly spaced initial y-coordinates of the rare cell. The x-coordinate is zero for all of them. We record the final y-coordinate at the outflow after one pass of the chamber in each of the 10 simulations with different random seeding of red blood cells. This way we obtain 100 final rare cell positions.

We denote the vector of initial positions $[p_1, \ldots, p_{10}]$, the vector of final positions $[q_1, \ldots, q_{100}]$ and the corresponding vector of weights after i iterations $\mathbf{w} = [w_1^i, \ldots, w_{100}^i]$, which is set to $[1, \ldots, 1]$ at the beginning. After each hypothetical rare cell pass of the simulated chamber, we redistribute the vector of weights using the simulation results. For each final position q_j, we look for the closest initial positions p_{upper} and p_{lower}, such that $p_{upper} > q_j > p_{lower}$. We compute the weights $\alpha = (p_{upper} - q_j)/(p_{upper} - p_{lower})$ and $(1 - \alpha)$. We then add the weight 0.1α to each of the 10 rare cell trajectories starting from p_{lower} and $0.1(1 - \alpha)$ to each of the 10 rare cell trajectories starting from p_{upper}. The new weights $\mathbf{w}_{new}$ are then obtained as $\mathbf{w}_{old}$ multiplied by the obtained weights of rare cell trajectories in this iteration.

The final weights represent the distribution of rare cell positions at the end of the simulation chamber (in x direction). We have repeated this process N_{pass} times for the four column diameters and obtained the distributions depicted in Figure 6.7. Note, they show two peaks due to the symmetric nature of the problem.

As we can see, with increasing number of RBCs in the simulation, the rare cell distributions are slightly *wider*. This means that the red blood cells have some impact on the rare cell trajectory although this impact is not very pronounced with hematocrit up to 10%, as can be seen in Table 6.2.

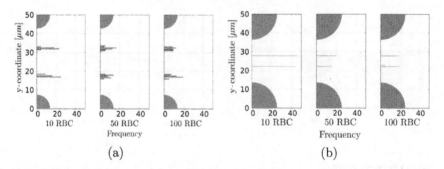

FIGURE 6.7: Histogram of typical rare cell positions between two obstacles for $N_{pass} = 400$: (a) $r = 7\mu m$, (b) $r = 13\mu m$.

n_{cell}	$r = 7$		$r = 9$		$r = 11$		$r = 13$	
	Ht	P	Ht	P	Ht	P	Ht	P
10	2.79	1.43	2.92	13.75	3.09	38.12	3.33	76.48
50	5.42	1.78	5.67	12.54	6.00	36.59	6.46	77.33
100	8.71	2.01	9.10	12.13	9.64	34.93	10.38	73.38

TABLE 6.2: Capture rates, radii in μm.

6.4.7   Interpretation of results

We have calculated the capture rate over the N_{pass} passes of the periodic chamber as

$$P = \sum_{i=1}^{N_{pass}} \sum_{j=1}^{100} w_j^i P_j, \qquad (6.7)$$

where P_j is calculated using (6.5). We have examined 10 different rare cell starting trajectories and for each of them, 10 different random RBC seedings. Thus we have 100 trajectories for each combination of the column radius and cell count.

In order to verify that the calculated capture rates correspond to those we could obtain from long simulations, we have run two different seedings for 10 RBCs and two for 50 RBCs. We have compared their capture rates with rates calculated using our new method and confirmed that up to the variation due to the fact that the simulation shows one particular setup while the calculation uses an average of several setups, the capture rates are comparable.

Overall, the calculated capture rates are slightly higher than the rates coming from long simulations. The reason for this is that when the rare cell slides along the micropost in the simulation - no matter how close - in the calculation we can only use the lowest or highest seeding position, which gives us less contact. From this we conclude that in our setup we can deduce the rare cell behavior even from short simulations.

Our simulations show that both column radius and hematocrit influence the trajectories of rare cells. We observe that an increase in column radius increases the capture rate quadratically. Further detailed analysis of the results reveals an interesting observation: For obstacle radius $7\mu m$, the capture rate increases with increased RBC count from 50 to 100 while for other radii, capture rate decreases. One possible explanation is that there is more physical space available in the microchannel with $r = 7\mu m$. At this radius, RBCs push the rare cell towards the obstacle which results in an increased capture rate but they still have enough physical space so as not to get between the rare cell and the obstacle. Different behavior can be seen at obstacle radii 9, 11 and 13 μm. Here, although RBCs push the rare cell towards the obstacle, they have less space and they get between the rare cell and the obstacle. This contributes to a slight linear decrease of the overall capture rate with an increasing number of RBCs.

6.5 Collision rates and deterministic lateral displacement in POAs

Recently, computational modeling has been successfully used for determination of collision rates in periodic obstacle arrays. To determine suitable geometry, a strategy called geometrically enhanced differential immunocapture (GEDI) has been used in [75, 99, 166, 175]. Two-dimensional Navier-Stokes equations were solved to obtain the velocity profile of the fluid inside the device. Subsequently, particle advection simulations were performed to advect the cell positions inside the flow. This approach utilises a one-way interaction between fluid and cells: The fluid determines the cell flow but the cells do not affect the fluid back. The data obtained about the cell trajectories, their positions, cell orientations, etc., were used to analyse different geometries. Gleghorn and Smith in [76, 175] have specified the design parameters that induce high collision rates for all particles larger than a threshold size or selectively increase the collision frequencies for a narrow range of particle sizes within a polydisperse population.

It is however natural to expect that the cell concentration influences the collision rate of the cells and it is important to understand how. Experimentally, if we wanted to avoid this influence, we could dilute the cell suspension to the level at which no cell-cell collisions occur. This leads to processing of larger volumes and thus to longer processing times. This is disadvantageous, since a long processing time may have an adverse impact on the viability of circulating tumor cells [96]. Using a model such as the one described in this book, that accounts for cell-cell collisions, is a natural choice.

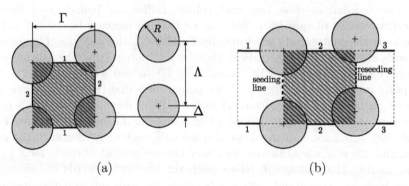

(a)   (b)

FIGURE 6.8: Schematics of periodic obstacle arrays and simulation setups. (a) Part of the array with periodic block indicated as a dashed region. The velocity fields at two lines marked by 1 are identical due to periodicity. The same holds for lines marked by 2. (b) A simulated periodic block is indicated as a dashed region and computational domain is bounded by a dashed line. In both experiments A and B, the cells that reach the reseeding line are moved and seeded at the seeding line.

6.5.1   Performing a simulation study

Dilute suspensions were thoroughly studied by [76, 175]. They have obtained collision rates by periodically repeating the streamlines of the flow. Before designing new simulations experiments, it is good to test the model to see whether we can reproduce the same results as the previously described experiments. For this we set up Experiment A, where the individual cells do not interfere and do not influence each others' trajectories by mutual collisions.

Microfluidic channels that contain periodic obstacle arrays are typically flat channels with their width and length much larger than their height. We model channels containing 100 columns of obstacles. Since the obstacle positions are periodic, we may consider only one repeating block. In Figure 6.8 (a), one such block is indicated as a dashed region. The size of this block is $150 \times 150 \times 30\mu m^3$. In all experiments, $\Gamma = \Lambda = 150\mu m$, $R = 50\mu m$. The radius of cells was set to $9\mu m$. The flow rate was set to the same value as in [76] to reproduce the results.

The one question that remains is how to set up the computational domain. The computational framework supports periodic boundary conditions. This is advantageous, since we would like to model a periodically repeating block - see Figure 6.8 (a). However, a closer look reveals that the two vertical boundaries denoted by 2 are shifted with a vertical offset Δ. Theoretically, it is indeed possible to set up such shifted boundary conditions (BC) in the lattice-Boltzmann model. This however requires extensive modification of the model implementation. To circumvent this issue, we can add additional channel length before and after the periodic box, so that the streamlines can adapt. In order to do that, we take our computational domain in x-direction to have 325 μm in length. This way, the fluid evolves into an almost shifted-periodic flow profile at the seeding and reseeding lines. The boundary conditions at inflow and outflow are set to periodic.

6.5.2 Parameter ranges and observed characteristics

Experiment A - Dilute suspension

We have seeded the cells uniformly at the left inflow starting with a cell touching the bottom-left obstacle and ending with a cell touching the top-left obstacle. The cell position is given by the position of its center. The seeding positions all have the x-coordinate 0, the z-coordinate 15 and the y-coordinate ranges from 59 to 91, incremented by 0.5 μm. Altogether, this results in 65 different seeding positions. For each seeding position, we have recorded the traces of the cell until its x-coordinate reaches Γ.

Given these 65 traces we can reconstruct the movement of the cell through the periodic obstacle array containing 100 columns. The y-coordinate of the cell at the end of the first trace defines the seeding position for the second trace, taking into account the offset Δ. Subsequently, the y-coordinate at the end of the second trace defines the seeding position for the third trace, etc. For higher accuracy, we have used interpolation between the neighboring traces.

This way we were able to simulate the movement of the cells through the periodic device. During the simulation, we have counted how many times the cell passed an obstacle and simultaneously we have counted whether during this passage the cell touched the obstacle. Then, a simple ratio of these two numbers gives us the collision-per-row frequency, denoted by CpR.

The obtained results were as expected. They are presented in Figure 6.9 (a). Comparison with results depicted in Figure 8a (right) in [76] shows that both results are identical. In both figures we can see that the most favorable geometry is at $\Delta/\Gamma_{opt} = 0.17$. With this experiment we have demonstrated that our model can successfully reproduce previous results.

In the range $\Delta/\Gamma \in (0, 0.17)$ the CpR is monotonically increasing, reaching its maximum at $\Delta/\Gamma_{opt} = 0.17$, which is the optimal ratio for maximizing the CpR. In the range $\Delta/\Gamma \in (0.17, 0.42)$ CpR varies, but basically, it gets only four different values: 0.25, 0.33, 0.4 and 0.5. In the range $\Delta/\Gamma \in (0.42, 0.5)$ the values of CpR gradually decrease from 0.5 to 0.2.

From these results we may conclude that there are two modes for typical cell trajectories: the colliding mode and the zig-zag mode. In the colliding mode, $\Delta/\Gamma \in (0, 0.17)$ and the cells pass the obstacles along the top of the obstacle and are further diverted up to pass again along the top of the next obstacle (with the exception of very few passes in the beginning of their trajectory through the obstacle array). In the zig-zag mode, $\Delta/\Gamma \in (0.17, 0.5)$

and the cells are sometimes diverted up to pass along the top of the next obstacle and sometimes are diverted down to pass along the bottom of the next obstacle. The concrete interplay between how often they are diverted up and down determines the actual CpR.

Experiment B - Low to middle density suspension

Natural questions may arise: Does the profile of CpR change when there are more cells inside the channel? Do mutual cell-cell collisions affect the CpR? In what way?

These questions have led us to set up another computational experiment.

We have performed a set of simulations for three different cell counts: $n_1 = 5, n_2 = 10, n_3 = 15$ cells, which correspond to the volume fractions of 3.5%, 6.9% and 10.4%

For each cell density $n_i, i = 1, 2, 3$, we have performed 76 long time simulations, one for each $\Delta = 0, 1, \ldots, 75 \mu m$. For each Δ, we have randomly seeded the corresponding number of cells between the seeding line and the reseeding line, avoiding the obstacles. Then we let the flow evolve and we have recorded the trajectories of individual cells. As soon as a cell has reached the reseeding line, we have moved it back to the seeding line while preserving its distance from the bottom obstacles. The simulations were long enough so that each cell passed the reseeding line at least 50 times in order to get correct statistical data.

We are aware that the flow pattern between the obstacles at the reseeding line is affected by the cells right before the reseeding of the cells. The flow at the seeding line however is not. This inaccuracy is negligible because the cells located at the reseeding line right before the reseeding follow the flow field and their velocity is almost identical compared to the velocity of the surrounding fluid in an empty channel after the flow completely evolves. The relative difference stays under 1%.

In Experiment B, we have obtained completely different results depicted in Figure 6.9 (b)–(d). With five cells in the channel, the cell-to-fluid ratio is only 3.5%. Even at such low cell density we have obtained different optimal Δ/Γ. Although the shape of the curve at Figure 6.9(b) resembles the shape from Figure 6.9(a), the optimal value has shifted from 0.17 to $\Delta/\Gamma_{opt} = 0.12$.

This can be explained by looking more closely at the cell trajectories. As we have pointed out before, in dilute suspensions at optimal $\Delta/\Gamma = 0.17$, the trajectory of the cell is in colliding mode: the cell touches the top of the obstacle after a few passes. From then on, the cell follows the top of the obstacle and is further diverted up towards the top of the next obstacle. The size of the cell and Δ ensure that the cell does not get below the next obstacle and that the trajectory does not change to the zig-zag mode.

In the experiment with cell-to-fluid ratio 3.5% and $\Delta/\Gamma = 0.17$, the cells sometimes collide with other cells and thus get pushed in an out-of-streamline direction. This direction is either up or down. While the direction up does not

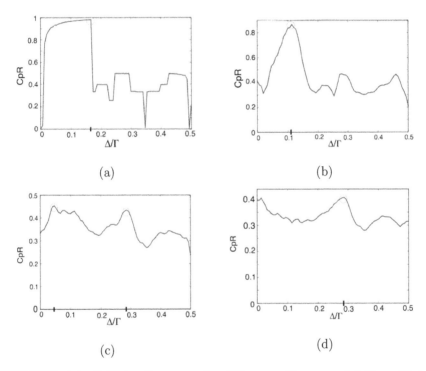

FIGURE 6.9: Collision frequency for different cell counts. (a) Very dilute solution. (b) Five cells, hematocrit 3.5%. (c) Ten cells, hematocrit 6.9%. (d) Fifteen cells, hematocrit 10.4%. Optimal values of Δ/Γ and CpR are indicated with thick tic marks and circles.

influence whether the cell remains in the colliding mode, the direction down can cause the cell to go below the obstacle and thus switch to zig-zag trajectory. This subsequently decreases the CpR. To ensure that such an occasional downward collision does not divert the cell below the next obstacle, Δ must be lower. Therefore the optimal Δ/Γ ratio decreases for 3.5% hematocrit.

This phenomenon however is not present at even higher hematocrits. With 10 cells and a 6.9% cell-to-fluid ratio, the situation is different. The highest CpR is reached for two values $\Delta/\Gamma_{opt} = 0.06$ and $\Delta/\Gamma_{opt} = 0.28$. With 15 cells and a 10.4% cell-to-fluid ratio, there is a single optimum at $\Delta/\Gamma_{opt} = 0.28$. We can clearly see from Figure 6.9 that the maximal CpR in these two cases reaches only 0.45 and 0.4, respectively.

This is caused by numerous cell-cell collisions causing the cells to be diverted below the obstacle too often. The cell simply never stays at the colliding mode for the whole course in the periodic obstacle array. From this behavior we can conclude that with higher cell-to-fluid ratio, cell trajectories are never in fully colliding mode. This is a very important observation because it suggests that with higher hematocrits one cannot expect too high CpR.

6.5.3   Interpretation of results

In this simulation study, we have seen that the collision frequency in periodic obstacle arrays strongly depends on the cell-to-fluid ratio. For very dilute suspensions where no mutual cell collisions occur, one can use particle advection simulations to determine optimal Δ/Γ. However for more detailed analysis for non-optimal values Δ/Γ a more detailed framework, such as the one described here, may give more accurate results.

For suspensions with cell-to-fluid ratio starting at 3.5%, one needs to account for mutual cell collisions. Our simulations showed significant differences when determining optimal Δ/Γ ratio for different suspension densities. Not only does the optimal value change, but the optimum may be reached at multiple values, as shown in Figure 6.9 (c).

The simulations further revealed that the cell trajectories in periodic obstacle arrays are in two modes: the colliding mode where the cell is always diverted up along the upper edge of the obstacles, and the zig-zag mode, where the cell is repeatedly diverted up and down.

In dilute suspensions and in suspensions with cell-to-fluid ratio at 3.5%, both modes occur and it is possible to determine the range of obstacle offset Δ/Γ, for which the cells follow the colliding mode. For suspensions with cell-to-fluid ratios at 6.9% and 10.4%, the cells never enter the colliding mode and remain in zig-zag mode. This means that collision frequency rapidly decreases in these cases.

6.6 Blood damage index

One of the quantities that needs to be minimized when developing new blood-contacting devices is the amount of shear-induced hemolysis. Among other factors, such hemolysis is a result of shear forces in flow, collisions with other blood cells and the contact with the device boundaries. There have been numerous attempts to quantify this kind of cell damage.

Hemolysis

Hemolysis is the rupturing - lysis - red blood cells. As a result, their inner fluid - cytoplasm - which is rich in hemoglobin, is released to the blood plasma. In addition to destroyed cells, the second negative effect is the free hemoglobin, which is toxic to vasculature and exposed tissues.

It has been shown that the lysis of red blood cells happens either when they are exposed to large shear stress over a short period of time (at the order of 1000 N/m^2 in several milliseconds) or by smaller stresses (at the order of 150 N/m^2) to which the cells are exposed for a longer time (over 100 seconds) [44]. The constant uniform shear stress has been linked to the undesirable free hemoglobin in the blood plasma [184] and this indicates that computer simulations can be very useful in the design of various devices where such damage would pose an issue.

Several approaches based on the power law equation have been proposed to calculate the amount of hemolysis [117], where the shear stress is integrated over the exposure time following the velocity streamlines. While these computations are fast, due to their simplicity, they cannot predict the magnitude of hemolysis very accurately [184].

Using a single-cell model such as the one described in this book, it is possible to obtain information on the possible cell damage of whole blood, stress on single blood cells and also incorporate and analyse the effect of cell-cell interactions [85]. It can be done using the cell damage index (CDI), which relies on the increase in local and global cell membrane areas.

The index is calculated as follows, illustrated in Figure 6.10: First a cumulative deviation of global area ($CDG_{cell_{ID}}$) is calculated for each cell:

$$CDG_{cell_{ID}} = \sum_i \frac{|S_i - S_0|}{S_0} \Delta t,$$

where S_i is the current global surface of the cell, S_0 is the original surface of the cell (in relaxed state) and $\frac{|S_i - S_0|}{S_0}$ is the current absolute relative change of global surface. The sum is computed for each cell in the monitored region of the channel with constant time steps Δt as illustrated in the following code snippet.

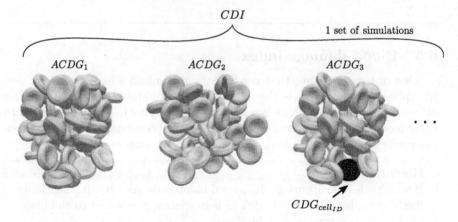

FIGURE 6.10: Scheme of relationships between CDI, $ACDG_{sim_{ID}}$ and $CDG_{cell_{ID}}$. Reprinted from [85] with permission [84].

```
# calculation of relative global area change for each cell:
relaxed_surface = cell.surface()
sum_of_relative_global_area_changes = 0
for i in range(0, max_timesteps+1):
    global_area_change = np.abs(cell.surface() - relaxed_surface)
    sum_of_relative_global_area_changes += \
    global_area_change*time_step/relaxed_surface
```

Next we compute the average cumulative deviation of global surface from all tracked cells in one simulation $ACDG_{sim_{ID}}$ as

$$ACDG_{sim_{ID}} = \frac{1}{n_{cell}} \sum_{cell_{ID}=1}^{n_{cell}} CDG_{cell_{ID}},$$

where n_{cell} is the number of cells in a simulation, for which we track $CDG_{cell_{ID}}$.

Finally, the CDI is calculated as an arithmetic mean of $ACDG_{sim_{ID}}$ from a set of simulations with the same channel geometry:

$$CDI = \frac{1}{N_{sim}} \sum_{sim_{ID}=1}^{N_{sim}} ACDG_{sim_{ID}},$$

where N_{sim} is the number of simulations in a set, for which we calculate the index. Each simulation starts with a random position of the cells.

While under large shear stress, the change in volumetric content of red blood cells in the whole blood does not have an effect on the hemolysis (basically, the cells get damaged with or without their friends nearby) [115], under lower stress, the cell-cell interactions have a major impact on the CDI [85], i.e. it does matter whether the cells come into contact with other cells or not.

Note that with the model introduced in this book, we could analyse the surface changes even on a finer scale, since we also have information about local area changes relative to their relaxed values.

6.7   Ventricular assist devices

There is an eminent interest in optimisation of *ventricular assist devices* (VADs). These are basically pumps that help blood to circulate in a body of patients suffering from heart failure. The schematic of such a pump is depicted in Figure 6.11. The pumping is done by a rotating impeller, which causes high shear stresses and consequently damage of red blood cells.

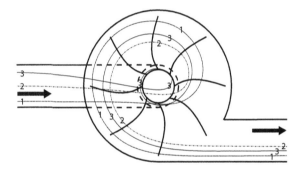

FIGURE 6.11: Scheme of a ventricular assist device. Blood enters the device through a central pipe and is propelled by rotating blades. Three different pathways for single cells are depicted. Pathway 3 represents movement with one extra rotation compared to pathways 1 and 2.

We devoted the previous section to quantification of cell damage using information on cell deformations in dense flows. This approach may be used in cases when the size of the device in consideration is small enough to be captured in one simulation. The number of cells in such a device is a limiting factor. A variant of this method may be used in cases when the device has sections that are periodically repeating. One can thus simulate only one section of the device reducing the number of cells to be simulated.

When an irregular device is in consideration, without any periodically re-peating parts, the problem must be approached differently. Other approaches for estimation of blood cell damage rely on macroscopic modeling of the whole blood as a uniform fluid. The macroscopic point of view allows for modeling of the whole device, however on a rather coarse scale, as we have mentioned in the previous section. The cell damage is then expressed as a time integral of the shear stress inside the device. Combining both of these approaches seems to profit from both scenarios. First, modeling the device macroscopically would give information about the shear stress that a cell feels while passing through the device. Then, this information can be fed into a single-cell model to mimic exactly the same local environment, which the cell is exposed to in the device. As a result, we have a single-cell deformation that is the same as it would be in the device. Consequently, one can further evaluate the amount of stress on the membrane, locate the highest stresses, determine locations in the device that add the most to the cell damage, etc.

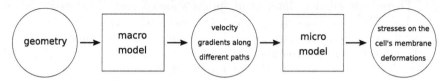

FIGURE 6.12: Workflow for modeling of mechanical stress on a membrane of RBC during its passage through a ventricular assist device.

The graphical representation of this process is depicted in Figure 6.12. The geometry of a VAD is inserted into a computational fluid dynamics software. There are numerous possibilities including commercial codes or open-source solutions. Such software may use macroscopic models for the turbulent flow based on Navier-Stokes equations or lattice-Boltzmann equations. In these models, the blood is treated as a homogeneous fluid.

A numerical solver of the macroscopic problem gives information about the velocity field in the device. Integrating this field gives the position in time of the fictitious particles that can be considered as cells driven by the flow. The movement of fictitious particles thus gives approximate trajectories of cells. The individual trajectories, of course, depend on the initial location of the particles entering the device. Once these trajectories are known, one can determine the velocity gradient along these trajectories as the main output of the macroscopic model.

Further, we can now continue with the microscopic model from Chapter 3. The idea is to simulate a small cubic volume around one cell such that the cell *feels* as if it was passing through a VAD. This can be achieved by setting suitable boundary conditions of the cubic box that result in the exact same velocity gradient as is locally in the VAD around this cell. In Section 4.3.2, we describe Couette flow with constant shear rate along the whole channel. Such flow may be generated by moving the top and bottom walls, see Figure 6.13 (a). In this case, the shear rate is induced along the z-direction and the velocity gradient is equal to

$$\nabla \mathbf{u} = \begin{pmatrix} \frac{\partial u_1}{\partial x} & \frac{\partial u_1}{\partial y} & \frac{\partial u_1}{\partial z} \\ \frac{\partial u_2}{\partial x} & \frac{\partial u_2}{\partial y} & \frac{\partial u_2}{\partial z} \\ \frac{\partial u_3}{\partial x} & \frac{\partial u_3}{\partial y} & \frac{\partial u_3}{\partial z} \end{pmatrix} = \begin{pmatrix} 0 & 0 & c \\ 0 & 0 & 0 \\ 0 & 0 & 0 \end{pmatrix}$$

Since the data from the macroscopic model contain general velocity field $\nabla \mathbf{u}$, we need to think of how to model such a gradient in the middle of the cubic box. The idea is to set the boundary conditions on all six cubic walls in such a way that the resulting flow inside the cube resembles the requested velocity field, see Figure 6.13 (b). The implementation of such boundary conditions may be tricky since one needs to ensure proper recalculation of the velocities on the boundary, bearing in mind the conservation of the mass. The initial experiments with this approach have been done in [180].

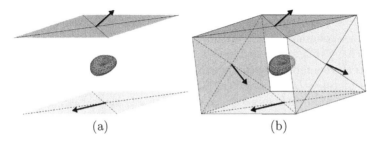

(a)   (b)

FIGURE 6.13: Cubic box around a cell and (a) Couette flow induced by moving the opposite walls and, (b) flow with more general velocity gradient induced by moving all walls of the cube.

After setting the correct boundary conditions, one can simulate the effect of the changing velocity field according to data obtained from macroscopic model. The boundary conditions cannot be varied within one run of the simulation in ESPResSo and therefore the velocity field must be approximated by a piecewise constant field. It is however possible to implement time-varying boundary conditions for further model improvements. The output from the microscopic model may be multifaceted. We can look at maximal elongation of the cell, on maximal stress on the membrane, we can follow parts of the membrane that are stressed constantly above a certain level, we can monitor how the total surface is being stretched. All of this information may help us assess the amount of deformation a single cell undergoes.

Moreover, we can use different data corresponding to different trajectories through the VAD. This way we can assess the trajectories that account for the most blood damage. By statistical sampling, we can evaluate the percentage of cells that have a large chance of being damaged by the shear stress. The previous two paragraphs describe the information that can be obtained for a single device design. If we use this data to go back in Figure 6.12 from the last circle to the first circle we can start the process of design optimisation for VAD.

The idea of simulating the immediate neighborhood of a cell during its passage through a microfluidic device is general enough to be used for any kind of devices, not only VADs. It can help in the design phase of device development and also in the analysis of cell behavior in the device.

6.8   Analysis of surface micro-roughness

In the previous sections we discussed several issues that involved particle-surface interactions. The surface may be walls of microfluidic device or surface of obstacles placed in flow. In this section, we focus on this kind of interaction again and discuss how a simulation model can help with analysis of the effect of the surface roughness on the mobility of microparticles. Blood cells of different sizes behave differently in blood flow. While the red blood cells are pulled towards the center of vessels thus forming a cell-free layer along the walls, the smaller platelets (thrombocytes) marginate toward the walls. This movement helps them fulfil their mission - to aggregate at places where repair is needed and cover any breaches in the vessel wall integrity. The shape and size of the platelets are different than those of RBCs.

The unactivated platelets are biconvex discoid structures with 2-$3\mu m$ in greatest diameter. In works that investigated the influence of a flat wall on platelet aggregation [133, 134], it has been shown that the platelet collision frequency and aggregation mechanics depend strongly on particle shape and distance from the bounding wall. However, surfaces are not always flat and the work [13] introduced micro-roughness of the surfaces at a length scale comparable to the sizes of spheroidal microparticles, which are a reasonable model of the unactivated platelets. While the work focuses on motion of individual platelets, in the future it would be instructive to study whole blood flows near micro-rough surfaces, because the motion of platelets could be influenced by the collisions with both RBCs and micro-bumps.

For now, using the computational model described in this book, it has been shown that the periodic roughness can quantitatively change the tumbling motion of the particles, Figure 6.14. The mechanical interaction of the particle with the micro-bumps repulses the particles from the surface and affects their mobility. The effect is strongly sensitive to the shape of the particle and is much more pronounced for oblate spheroids. The analysis has been done with rigid particles, since platelets in the non-activated state are known to be practically non-deformable.

The take-away message from this analysis is that in (microfluidic) devices where the adherence of platelets to walls is undesirable (e.g. implants), one of the ways to avoid it is an application of micro-rough surfaces as an anti-

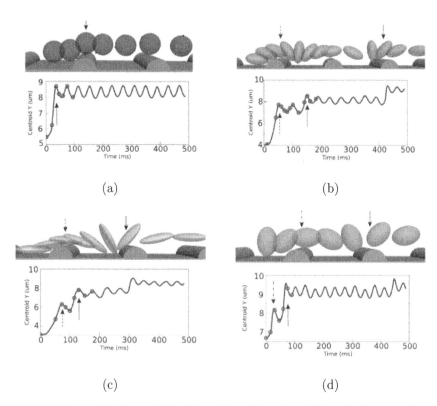

(a)

(b)

(c)

(d)

FIGURE 6.14: Each panel (a-d) consists of a series of simulation snapshots and the plot of y-coordinate of particle centroid vs. time. The red circles denote the respective moments of time, at which the snapshots were taken. The solid arrows mark moments of lift due to hitting the cylinder during flip-motion (panels b, c, d) and over-rolling (for panel a). The dashed arrows correspond to lift due to over-crawling (panels b, c). The dash-dotted arrow in panel d corresponds to over-hopping the obstacle. (Reprinted from [13] with permission [12].)

thrombotic coating. This mechanical solution would be especially useful in cases where the biological coating is problematic.

Chapter 7

Ideas for extension

7.1   Advantage of modular approaches or isolate cleverness

Consider UNIX, a powerful operating system that has many tiny command line routines. Outputs of many of them can be fed as inputs to many others. This works because each of them does a single thing and does it well. The features are efficient, well-defined and isolated. We can stack them up and create something bigger.

And our models should do the same. They should have clever and flexible building blocks that can be stacked and reused. An example of this is the force-based approach to elastic objects. Several new properties can be introduced using the force principles and we describe some of them in this chapter.

7.2   Rolling and adhesion of cells

There are two principal modes in which cell interacts with a wall: Either there is no biological activity between cell and the wall and the only effect of wall onto the cell is that it does not allow the cell to penetrate the wall. Alternatively, the surface of the wall is functionalised with proteins that react with surface proteins of the cell. They create bonds and this can cause cells to slow down or even to adhere to the surface.

The first case can be modeled by repulsive potentials in our model. Similarly to the cell-cell interaction described in Section 3.6, the potential keeps some very small distance between the particles of the cell mesh and the wall.

The second case is much more difficult to implement, but the force-based approach of our model allows us to define additional adhesion forces that mimic the creation and rupture of protein bonds.

7.2.1 Adhesion models

To investigate the rolling and adhesion of biological cells to walls, we must look at the biological background of the cell rolling. The membrane of a cell is often covered with protruding proteins. These are called receptors. The walls of the microchannel may be functionalised with a different type of proteins, these are called ligands. Ligands are mostly complementary to receptors and they both interact with each other by forming a tight bond. These bonds in fact form a sort of mechanical spring with a given stiffness and its own dynamics of creation and rupture.

During its journey through the microfluidic device, once the cell comes close enough to a functionalised wall, receptors and ligands start forming bonds slowing the motion of the cell down [178].

We have already mentioned adhesion of the cells in a simplified case. In Section 6.4 we have presented a model with lumped parameters for individual receptors and ligands. The procedure for grouping several sub-microscopic parameters into lumped parameters is described by relations (6.4) and (6.5).

Before a receptor and a ligand can form a bond, their physical locations need to be brought to a close vicinity. The physical distance (called capture radius r_0) allowing to form a bond is defined by the lengths of proteins forming receptors and ligands. When the receptor and the ligand are within this distance, an *encounter complex* has been formed. This does not automatically mean that a bond has been created. During the encounter phase, a bond between the receptor and the ligand can be created with a certain probability. Reversely, any bond can rupture with a certain probability during this time. The more the bond is stretched, the larger is the probability of the rupture. Eventually, as the cell rolls further and the distance between the receptor and the ligand grows above a certain threshold (denoted by critical bond length), the bond - if it still exists - breaks. Schematics of the bond creation and bond rupture are depicted in Figure 7.1.

The adhesion mechanism described above is based on bonds between the receptor site on a cell and the ligand site on a wall. Once the stiffness κ of such a bond is known, one can model this bond by putting a repulsive or attractive force at the corresponding mesh point. The computation of the adhesive forces acting on the end points of the bond is based on the harmonic spring. If a bond complex exists and the distance between the receptor position and the ligand position is l, then the magnitude of affinity force is computed from

$$F_{ad} = \kappa l.$$

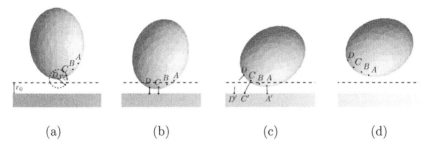

(a)   (b)   (c)   (d)

FIGURE 7.1: Schematics of bond formation using a cell with four highlighted boundary points - receptors - denoted by black points. (a) The distance of the cell to the surface is larger than the capture radius r_0. No encounter complex has been formed and thus no bonds can be created. (b) Three boundary points B, C and D are within the capture radius. For these points, an encounter complex has been created. The stochastic nature of the bond creation resulted in the formation of two bonds with receptor positions C and D, while there was no bond created for receptor B. Corresponding ligand positions at the wall are indicated by C' and D'. (c) As possible due to the stochastic nature of the bond creation, there still has not been any bond formed for receptor B. Receptor C is now out of the capture radius, however, the bond CC' has not reached the critical length l_{max} for the rupture and the stochastic nature of bond dissociation has not caused the bond to rupture yet. Receptor D is out of the capture radius. It had reached the critical bond length l_{max} and the bond has ruptured. (d) The cell has moved away from the wall and all the bonds have ruptured.

There are other possibilities. For example one can assume the resting length l_0 and the force can be proportional to the positive prolongation and zero otherwise

$$F_{ad} = \begin{cases} \kappa(l - l_0) & \text{for } l > l_0, \\ 0 & \text{otherwise.} \end{cases}$$

We use the former simpler implementation showing that it is sufficient in our simulations.

Dissociation and association dynamics

During the time the encounter complex exists, it can react to creation of a bond with the on-rate k_{on}. This is represented by the probability P_{on} of bond formation during time step Δt. Any bond can rupture into the encounter complex with the off-rate k_{off} with dissociation probability P_{off} over time Δt. Association and dissociation probabilities are expressed as

$$P_{on} = 1 - e^{-k_{on}\Delta t}, \qquad P_{off} = 1 - e^{-k_{off}\Delta t}.$$

While the association on-rate is constant, the dissociation rate k_{off} may depend on several quantities. In [106] they define

$$k_{off} = k_0 e^{\frac{F_{ad}}{F_d}} = k_0 e^{\frac{\kappa l}{F_d}}, \tag{7.1}$$

where k_0 is the dissociation rate at zero pulling force, F_{ad} is the magnitude of adhesion force on the bond and F_d is the detachment force scale. This model for k_{off} has been demonstrated to properly describe the dissociation process for selectin bonds in the high force regime [27].

The problem with this model is determination of its individual parameters. Not only does one need to measure k_0, the dissociation rate of proteins at zero pulling force, the detachment force scale is given by relation

$$F_d = \frac{k_B T_a}{x_c},$$

where k_B is the known Boltzmann constant, T_a is also the known variable ambient temperature but x_c is to-be-determined case-by-case variable reactive compliance that has to be measured for each different protein [5]. The measurements of k_0 and x_c are not trivial, are protein dependent and require advanced laboratory equipment.

There is thus a question whether we can somehow get rid of these parameters.

Aggregate bond
The idea is that we do not model each individual bond, but rather we group several bonds and treat them as one *aggregate bond*. This way, the effect of multiple bonds on the membrane is replaced by the effect of one aggregate bond. The properties of multiple bonds are thus averaged. The question is what parts of the model should be omitted. The form of the

adhesion force will be unchanged. Grouping of multiple bonds will result in one aggregate bond with a higher stiffness constant.

The stochastic nature of bond formation will also be affected by bond grouping. We may assume that the probabilities can be computed by the same relations with just different association and dissociation constants.

The main difference will be in computation of the dissociation constant. In relation (7.1), the only variable is length of the bond l. If considering one aggregate bond as replacement of multiple bonds, one can assume that the averaged length will be close to a cell-wall minimal distance [106]. As a result, it is promising to consider k_{off} to be constant.

The model from [106] includes the dependence of k_{off} on the magnitude of the force exerted on the bond. We consider a simplified model when k_{off} is a fixed constant and we show that this simplified model can capture the important mesoscopic behavior caused by cell adhesion.

7.2.2 Calibration of model parameters

The simplified model of aggregate bond cannot use parameters of physical bonds such as bond stiffness, for example. We need to determine those parameters from available experiments. We can start from values obtained from biological experiments listed in [106].

In the following two experiments we would like to show that our simplified model can capture important behavior during the adhesion processes.

In the first experiment we test whether our model can capture statistical properties of velocity profile. We track the velocity of individual cells during the adhesion movement. The movement of the adherent cell is much slower than that of the un-adherent cell due to bonds between ligands and receptors. Since the bonds on a cell in the downstream break and bonds in the upstream are continuously created, the cell rolls on the surface. The velocity of the cell itself however randomly oscillates according to how often bonds break and how often they are created again. Because of the random nature of bond creation, every simulation run gives a different velocity profile. However, one can look at the mean value and the standard deviation and compare the simulated movement with the measured data for real cells.

The second experiment reveals that our model can capture the dependence of cell velocity on the different fluid shear stresses. Namely, the question is whether one parameter set gives the same values of averaged velocity of the cell for different fluid shear stresses.

The model was tested and validated in simple shear flow. A microfluidic chamber was set up with height $h = 10\mu m$ with the upper wall moving in x-direction with velocity v_{wall}. This movement induces Couette flow in the chamber. The velocity of the fluid thus depends on the z-coordinate only and is constant in each plane parallel to the xy plane. The velocity in Couette flow reads as $v(z) = \frac{z}{h}v_{wall}$. The shear stress τ of the fluid in this type of flow can be expressed as $\tau = \mu \frac{dv(z)}{dz} = \mu \frac{v_{wall}}{h}$. Since the shear stress is constant in the whole channel, we also have this value for the wall shear stress. The fluid properties are those of water at temperature $T = 37°C$, $\rho_f = 1000 kgm^{-3}$, $\mu = 7.22 \times 10^{-4} Pas$.

Statistical properties

In [5], the authors performed laboratory experiments and obtained the rolling velocity of the cells, which our model can reconstruct. In Figure 7.2 we can see the measured velocities depicted by diamonds and the velocities obtained from our model depicted by squares. The parameters of our simplified model can be found in Table 7.1. Note that we were able to set the model parameters in such a way that both velocity profiles have the same mean value.

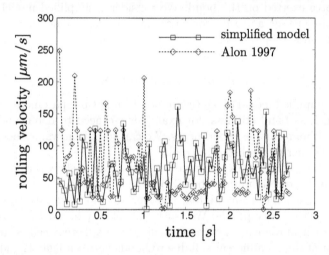

FIGURE 7.2: Velocity reconstruction over the time period of $3s$. The mean value of experimental data from [5] is the same as the mean value for the simulated velocity from our simplified model.

	Statistical properties	Dependence on shear stress
κ	0.08	0.14, 0.15
k_{on}	10^5	10^5
k_{off}	10^5	10^2

TABLE 7.1: Parameters of the simplified model for two experiments.

Dependence on fluid shear stress

In [46], the authors investigated the mechanics of leukocyte adhesion to endothelial cells using in vitro side-view flow assay. The authors showed how the

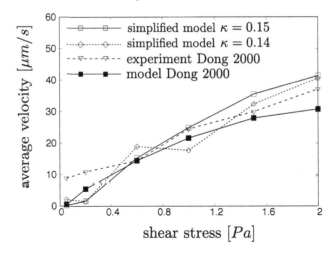

FIGURE 7.3: The averaged velocity of the cell over a certain time period depends on the wall shear stress. Both experimental and model data from [46] are shown. Our simplified model approximates the experimental data well for values $\kappa = 0.14, 0.15$.

averaged velocity of the cell depends on shear stress. We demonstrate that we are able to capture this dependence. The experiment was performed for shear stresses ranging from 0 to $2Pa$, for each stress we tracked the movement of the cell and we computed the averaged velocity over the time $1ms$. The results are presented in Figure 7.3.

7.3 Cell with a nucleus

So far, we have been mostly talking about modeling red blood cells. Highly elastic human red blood cells, whose one well-known characteristic is that they do not have a nucleus. Along with other organelles, it is expelled during the maturation process in the bone marrow [15]. This is presumably to gain space for more hemoglobin - an iron-containing protein whose function is to bind, transport and release oxygen. Even though not present in erythrocytes, the nucleus is an essential part of many other cells. It carries the genetic material and controls the cell by regulating the gene expression. It is a dense, roughly spherical organelle and a prominent feature of cells that have it.

The computational approaches to modeling cells with nuclei have been used in [25, 161] for CTCs and WBCs.

The model described in this book is general enough that one might consider also using it for cells other than RBCs. And this opens up a question how to model their nuclei.

Naturally, we start with a triangulation of the whole cell and represent the membrane like we have done so far. Then we can take a second triangulation, this time of a smaller sphere, and enclose it in the first one. If we just stopped here, these two membranes would behave independently and soon we would see their intersection and eventually even the nucleus leaving the cell. Putting aside some more or less catastrophic scenarios when this might happen, we would like the nucleus to remain inside and ideally influence the movement of the whole cell in such a way as the biological nucleus does. Therefore we must include some interactions between the membrane discretisation points to keep it in place.

There are basically two paths to explore, since in the model, we have two types of interactions: bonded and non-bonded. Bonded interaction is a relation between specific points: e.g. each stretching bond is an interaction between two points of an edge. Each bending bond is an interaction shared among four points that form the two triangles that share a common edge. If there is a change in the angle between these two triangles, all four points are affected. Volume force relies on a bonded interaction, too, even though this one is global. All points of the triangulation are *in the relationship*, because the volume of the object depends on all of their positions and thus all of them influence the volume force assigned at a single point. Compare this to non-bonded interaction. As the name suggests, this is not a bond between specific particles, but rather an interaction between each pair of particles of the given type. An example is a cell-cell interaction. We know that the two cells that come into proximity should repel each other (we describe the details of how this is done in Section 3.6), but we can specify a general rule:

If a particle of type 1 and a particle of type 2 get closer than the cutoff distance, do something.

Assuming that all triangulation nodes of one cell are of type 1 and all nodes of the other cell are of type 2, it does not matter where or how these two cells approach each other, they are going to do something about it locally.

Let us look at the bonded interactions first. They would imply defining bonds between some, maybe all, points in the nucleus mesh and some, maybe all, points of the outer membrane mesh. These would be specified at the beginning of the simulation, essentially joining the two meshes into one, and the connectivity of such joined mesh would remain fixed, see Figure 7.4 (a). These connecting bonds can be of the stretching type. They have to be soft enough so that the nucleus does not deform when the membrane is subjected to deformation, but stiff enough that the nucleus does not move much inside the membrane.

The following code snippet shows how to set up a cell with a nucleus using bonded interactions. First we create two spheres with the same center but

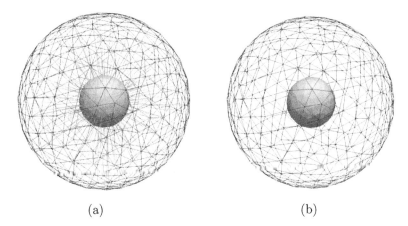

(a)   (b)

FIGURE 7.4: Two approaches to modeling a nucleus in a cell: (a) Using bonded interactions, and (b) using non-bonded interactions.

different radii. The inner sphere might have stiffer elastic coefficients and also possibly a larger mass. Then we define a small constant in radians that controls how many bonds a point of the nucleus will form with the outer membrane. For each point of the nucleus triangulation we use the three neighbors to calculate an approximate outer normal vector. Using the formula for angle between two vectors, we identify those points of the membrane triangulation, which are close enough to the outer normal. With these we create bonds. The small angle should be selected in such a way (with respect to the density of the triangulations) that there are between zero and three bonds per point of the nucleus, with not many zeroes and not many threes. The ideal situation would be if each point had exactly one bond. The bonds can be visualised in ParaView the same way as the stretching bonds on the surface.

```
# creating bonds between membrane and nucleus
small_angle = np.pi/15
lines = []
pairs = []
for p in nucleus.mesh.points:
    neighbors = nucleus.mesh.neighbors[p.id]
    normal = neighbors.outer_normal()
    lengthNormal = oif.norm(normal)
    pPos = p.get_pos()
    for pMembrane in membrane.mesh.points:
        pMembranePos = pMembrane.get_pos()
        tmpConnection = pMembranePos - pPos
        tmpDist = oif.norm(tmpConnection)
        angle = np.arccos(np.dot(tmpConnection,normal)/(tmpDist * \
```

```
lengthNormal))
if angle < small_angle:
    harmonicInter = HarmonicBond(k=0.05, r_0=tmpDist)
    system.bonded_inter.add(harmonicInter)
    p.part.add_bond((harmonicInter, pMembrane.part_id))
    tmplist = [pPos[0], pPos[1], pPos[2], pMembranePos[0], \
    pMembranePos[1], pMembranePos[2]]
    tmppair = [p.id, pMembrane.id]
    lines.append(tmplist)
    pairs.append(tmppair)
```

Since the approach that we have shown here is purely phenomenological (this is true both for bonded and non-bonded versions), the specific types of bonds that we use (e.g. non-linear stretching, harmonic or FENE in bonded and soft-sphere or membrane-collision in non-bonded version), do not matter as long as we can recover the desired behavior.

FENE vs. harmonic potential

FENE (Finite Extensible Non-linear Elastic) - Non-linear potential frequently used in spring models of long-chained polymers.

Harmonic - Quadratic potential used for deriving a potential energy function for a molecule.

Both of these potentials have minimum at the spring equilibrium distance and their graphs branch symmetrically upward on both sides of the minimum. The difference between them is that the FENE potential has a maximal extension/compression.

The second approach means defining a non-bonded interaction, between particles of the nucleus and particles of the outer membrane, Figure 7.4 (b). Obviously, it should be repulsive so that it keeps the nucleus inside the cell. The cutoff for this interaction should be set carefully. It cannot be too small, because then the nucleus would bounce inside the cell. But it also cannot be very large because then we would have all the outer points acting on all the inner points and the conflicting forces could lead to numerical instabilities. The sweet spot is around $r_M - r_n$, where r_M is the radius of the outer membrane and r_n is the radius of the nucleus. How do these two approaches compare? We can look at passage of a cell with nucleus through a narrow opening. This kind of investigation is done both in biological [24] and simulation [25], mainly to consider mechanisms of CTCs entering tissues and forming metastases.

So in principle, even though the model was primarily developed for red blood cells, this shows that it can also be extended to cells with nucleus. What has not been shown here, is the proper calibration of the membrane-nucleus interactions so that it corresponds to the biological behavior. Only after that can this kind of extension be used for examining the behavior of nucleated cells in simulations.

One thing to keep in mind for such calibration is the types of meshes used.

For the purposes of having the correct friction coefficient, even though we have just one cell, the two triangulations should be treated as two separate objects and thus their densities or average edge lengths should be approximately the same (see Section 3.5.2). As a consequence, the spheres will not have the same number of nodes and therefore there will (most likely) be nodes on the membrane surface that are not directly connected to the nucleus.

7.4   Solid objects

Modeling of a non-deformable object may be approached by various ways. One approach - a very simple one, when you have a model of a deformable object in hand - is to make the deformable object very stiff. This spares you the difficulties of creating a new model, but in fact, you are using a too complex model by allowing for deformability and at the same time restricting this deformability. There is another approach, using the same discretisation of the object's surface. It implements virtual sites [7]. These are the usual particles that are used to compose the membrane mesh, however with the one exception that their position, orientation and velocity are not obtained from the integration of Newton's equations of motion (3.11). Instead, these quantities are calculated from the position and orientation of another particle in the simulation. This non-virtual particle should be located at the center of mass of the rigid body and should carry the mass and inertial tensor of the complete body. The position and orientation of this center particle are obtained from the integration of Newton's equation, just as any other normal particle. The virtual sites that give the shape and interactions of the rigid body are placed relative to the position and orientation of the center particle and forces acting on them are translated back to forces and torques acting on the center particle, Figure 7.5. The force acting on the virtual site is copied to the center particle. In addition, the component of the force, which is orthogonal to the vector connecting the center of mass and virtual site, creates a torque on the center of mass. Using these forces and torques, Newton's equations can be integrated for the center of mass of the rigid bodies along with those for all the other non-virtual particles in the system. The subsequent positions and velocities of the virtual sites on the object's surface are then computed from the position of the center particle, its rotation velocity and the relative positions of virtual sites to the center particle. Using virtual sites, the raspberry model may be used for solid objects [41, 64].

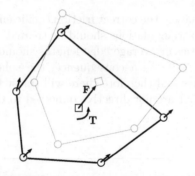

FIGURE 7.5: Virtual sites demonstrated in 2D. Two subsequent snapshots (black and grey) of one body are depicted. Virtual sites (black circles) have a fixed relative position against the center-of-mass particle (black square). Forces (small black arrows) acting on the surface in virtual points are transferred to the center-of-mass particle summing up to total force **F** and total torque **T**. Under the influence of **F** and **T**, the center-of-mass particle (black square) is moved and rotated into a new position (grey square). New positions of virtual sites (grey circles) are computed so that they keep the same relative position against the now rotated center-of-mass particle.

7.5 Movement of cell clusters (emboli)

Red blood cells sometimes form clusters. These often take the form of rouleaux - essentially stacks, in which the cells touch each other by their round *faces*. These kinds of aggregates have been computationally investigated in, e.g. [123]. Here we would like to talk about clusters of different kinds of cells. Both single cells and cell clusters (emboli) have been observed in the blood of patients with cancer. This behavior is not well understood, which is a good opportunity for computational investigation of how cell stiffness and cluster formation influence the cell transport.

The behavior of various individual particles in different types of flow has been investigated in, e.g. [34, 62]. A preliminary computational study with the aim to compare the spatio-temporal differences in the trajectories of various cell clusters has been performed by [20]. In it, the cell clusters (emboli) are composed of two or three individual cells that adhere to one another by classical harmonic potential

$$F(r) = \frac{1}{2}K(r - R)^2,$$

where r is the current bond length, $R = 0.5$ (in μm) is relaxed length of the bond and K is harmonic coefficient.

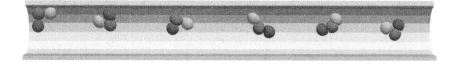

FIGURE 7.6: Cell cluster migrating towards the center of the pipe channel.

The simulation study considered multiple configurations, including different cluster shapes and orientations, Figure 7.6. The preliminary conclusions are that larger stiffness results in faster cluster rotation, and this rotation rate is dependent on the distance to the vessel wall. More investigation is needed, however, it is already clear that the presented model and its implementation can also be used for the investigation of cell clusters.

Chapter 8

Dreaming up the future

In this chapter we let our imagination run free. While in the previous chapters, we have relied on what is known and we have carefully added step-by-step building blocks on top of that to show how to build computational models, here we allow leaps, gaps, optimistic speculations and even a pinch of fiction here and there. This chapter is meant as an inspiration about where the cell modeling could lead and what it could be a part of in the future.

More than a hundred years ago, David Hilbert had presented 23 then-open problems that significantly shaped 20th century mathematics. Many of them have been resolved, but a few stubbornly continue to resist to this day.

In a similar fashion, at the beginning of this millennium, Joseph Hoffman summarised eight open areas for blood cell discoveries [94]. These pertained to both human and non-human red blood cells, considered questions both at molecular and cell scales and asked mostly about various mechanisms causing processes and properties of red cells. Some of these questions have partially been answered in the last few years, but overall, they still remain a challenge. Unlike Hilbert's problems, we would argue that with the increasing rate of progress in biosciences, none of these questions will remain without a satisfying answer for a century.

Hoffman's open areas for blood cell discoveries

1. What are the determinants of red cell shape? What is the precise structural/mechanical basis for the biconcave shape of the normal human red cell?

2. What is the high resolution structure of the red cell plasma membrane and how do the membrane properties depend on this structure?

3. What molecular mechanisms underlie the plasma membrane events associated with hemolysis of human red blood cells?

---

4. What are the genetic mechanisms responsible for the determination of red cell characteristics?

5. What are the regulatory mechanisms that determine a single red cell's volume?

6. What are the events responsible for removal of nuclei during the maturation process of human RBCs?

7. What determines the metabolic structure and function of red cells?

8. What are the genetic mechanisms involved in differentiation of stem cells into erythrocytes?

Sequencing complete genomes was a major step in bringing computational and algorithmic approaches to biological problems. With the computational power increasing, public databases of data made available and improvement of machine learning algorithms that can uncover relationships and build predictive models from observations, we already see further steps towards genetic fortune telling. Even in situations when we do not have sufficient explanation of the mechanisms that drive the outcome, by connecting enough dots among the observations, bioinformatics can undeniably improve the lives of many people. We have seen this, for example, in screening for *BRCA* gene mutations and subsequent preventative steps against breast cancer.

In the future, patient-specific treatment will also be available due to the computational power and models, as well. A patient-specific blood sample could be simulated and its response to various stimuli analysed, such as response to various versions of treatment for blood diseases before they are prescribed and subsequent selection of the best treatment options. Models could factor in an individual's age, diet, family history, environmental factors that influence the body's functions, possible side effects of drugs, etc.

Similar to Silicon Valley as a cradle of technological innovation, very likely there will be another cradle related to bio start-ups. As bluntly pointed out in the science fiction book [181], it is very unlikely that this bio-valley would be in California. While the technological and computational power is available there, the general US climate is not very welcoming to radical biological breakthroughs. On the one hand, this is good. Tinkering with the human genome, producing new organisms and playing with life matter in general should be approached with extreme caution because there could be unexpected irreversible consequences. Yet the realities in America make it more likely that the cutting-edge synthetic biological research will be done elsewhere. China has already started human CRISPR (gene editing) clinical trials and south-east Asia in general seems much more favorable.

What would be useful? Synthetic cells would be extremely useful. If we could produce good enough blueprints, e.g. high-fidelity models, cells could be printed by molecular nano-printers. Print enough blood cells, combine them with an artificial blood plasma and the increasing need for blood transfusion, as our population ages and demand is predicted to outpace supply, could be met. Synthesising other cells with their ability to grow and reproduce could be a clue to the throughput issues.

3D tissue bioprinting is almost available nowadays. The technologies that are needed for printing small pieces of tissue are already available. In these synthetic tissues, the cells can be organized in a fashion very similar to natural tissue. Simulations of cell behavior in the process of printing and cell interactions as they are assembled can aid in the development of these techniques and prototyping of various printers. The continuation of this trend could lead to growing new organic limbs or organs for people who miss or have lost their own. Models could certainly help with personalizing transplants and improving outcomes.

For example to enable the electronic-skin-based vision, the adaptation of soft biological tissue to external stimuli must be perfectly understood. Several models of soft biological tissue adaptation have been presented in [72]. The engineering of such devices leads to the prototypes of e-skins able to *see* things and to replace the potentially damaged retina [39]. But why stop here? Once a bridge between retina and the brain is understood, the e-skin may be placed anywhere on the body and thus people could *see* with their skin.

From here, the natural (and dangerous) next step is biofacturing. What if we do not want to limit ourselves to cells and parts of known organisms? Entirely newly designed bioproducts could be created: manufactured food or drugs tailored specifically to meet an individual's needs, cells that could battle specific diseases, bacteria that could help us decrease environmental pollution... the possibilities are endless, but all of them would heavily rely on biophysically realistic models enabled by future simulation tools and high-performance computing capabilities.

Ethical issues

While in a brainstorming session, such as this one, we can just let our ideas fly in any direction; in practice, these are certainly topics that need to be thought through extremely carefully. Ethical issues need to be considered. One thing is to change somatic cells and treat an individual organism. Quite another is to change germ cells and create and release a change that can propagate to new generations. These are issues already being discussed among the geneticists and others and will become more and more relevant with the increasing capabilities of biosciences.

On the one hand, we have the creation of new things, on the other is removal of those things that kill us. The 2016 Nobel Prize in chemistry was awarded to three scientists who discovered how to build nanomachines out of a chain of atoms. These light powered nanomachines - few specific molecules bound together - are engineered to be sensitive to specific proteins located on specific types of cells. They target these cells and kill them.

The damage done to cells was observed indirectly. Since there is a three-orders-of-magnitude length scale difference between the cell and the nanomachine, (today) it is not possible to observe both at the same time. The observation of cells showed membranes behaving as if they had so many hydrophilic pores - essentially holes - that they were irreversibly too damaged for the cells to live. Obviously, we would not want to do this to healthy cells, but the same thing happened when the nanomachines were unleashed on cancerous prostate cells.

Now imagine that their cell selection was reliable and could be trusted. It would open a field of nano-surgery, where we would not have to go after tumors and their metastases, but we could evict cancer from the body cell-by-cell. Taken one step further, consider an *inoculation-like* dose given preventively that patrols our bodies and kills the cells that turn cancerous before they can cause any damage. This way the nano-machines act as sensors and surgeons, but other logical steps would be to go into targeted drug delivery [1].

The big *if* here is the reliability and we are back to modeling. While an enormous amount of testing would have to be done with live cells and then tissues, it would be very helpful to accurately model the nanomachine-cell interaction in the design process.

And again, why stop here? What if these small surgeons were *intelligent*? Maybe not the nanomachines themselves since they are too small to contain enough information, but some cell-like vessels carrying these nanomachines that would contain genetic-like programs. Based on what the cell-vessels and their sensors encounter, they produce and release suitable nanomachines, observe the outcome and learn - an artificial immune system. This would need to be very carefully designed and computationally and biologically tested.

Even if these wild ideas do not become reality, similar to the report [145], we predict that computing will assume an increasing role in the working lives of nearly all biologists. Already today we see that a lot of discovery and advancement in biosciences is either directly done with or supported with computing and computational information processing. We expect this trend to continue and even grow further. It is very likely that various hybrid systems will emerge, where the (blood) cell modeling as we have introduced it in this book and its future generations will be one part of a larger model. For such synthesis of models, possibly across scales and approaches, it is likely that a common input/output biological data format or standard will crystallise, similar to json and xml available today.

To conclude, we return to the beginning and close the circle. Models are ultimately judged by their ability to make predictions - about future outcomes and about variables inaccessible to measurements. Simulations take over where analysis ends. But despite their power, models are not the goal. They capture only the essence of reality, not the full details and are tools to increase understanding and gain insight. Any answers they give need to be treated as hypotheses, tested and validated. Nevertheless, this does not diminish them. Models are tools that give us unprecedented possibilities to look and discover. Use them wisely.

Appendix A

Force- and torque-free bending modulus

A.1   Four-point interaction

Assume an interaction that serves to preserve an angle between two neighboring triangles in a spring network. The basic principle widely used is to apply forces to the vertices increasing the angle in case that the current angle is smaller than the one to be preserved, or the opposite forces otherwise. Clearly, such forces will be applied out-of-plane and it is natural to apply them perpendicularly to the triangles. This choice leaves us with the scenario depicted in Figure A.1. Here, two triangles ABC and ABD have common edge AB and they enclose angle θ. Denote θ_0 the angle to be preserved and assume $\theta > \theta_0$. The forces to be applied thus have directions as depicted in Figure A.1. The forces $\mathbf{F}_A, \mathbf{F}_B^1$ and $\mathbf{F}_C^1$ are applied to triangle ABC and $\mathbf{F}_D, \mathbf{F}_B^2$ and $\mathbf{F}_C^2$ are applied to triangle ABD.

The magnitudes of the forces are in principle free to choose in order to

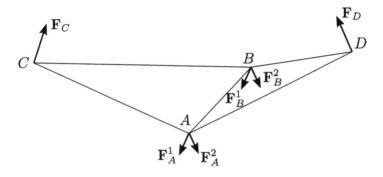

FIGURE A.1: Two adjacent triangles with bending forces.

decrease the angle between triangles. There are however two basic physical principles: without any external force, the object must conserve its momentum and angular momentum. In other words, the object should not start moving or rotating by itself. When modeling the elastic behavior of an object by spring networks, this translates to the force-free and torque-free conditions for all elastic forces.

To conform on the force-free condition for each triangle, the following must be valid

$$\mathbf{F}_A^1 + \mathbf{F}_B^1 = -\mathbf{F}_C \quad \text{and} \quad \mathbf{F}_A^2 + \mathbf{F}_B^2 = -\mathbf{F}_D.$$

These conditions are equivalent to choosing two factors k and l and to assign

$$\mathbf{F}_A^1 = -k\mathbf{F}_C, \quad \mathbf{F}_B^1 = -(1-k)\mathbf{F}_C \quad \mathbf{F}_A^2 = -l\mathbf{F}_D, \quad \mathbf{F}_B^2 = -(1-l)\mathbf{F}_D.$$

The directions of $\mathbf{F}_D$ and $\mathbf{F}_C$ can be expressed in terms of vector product of triangle edges. To allow for scaling of forces let us introduce scaling factors c and d and denote

$$\mathbf{F}_C = c(\mathbf{A} - \mathbf{C}) \times (\mathbf{B} - \mathbf{C}) \quad \text{and} \quad \mathbf{F}_D = d(\mathbf{B} - \mathbf{D}) \times (\mathbf{A} - \mathbf{D}). \quad \text{(A.1)}$$

For now, we do not discuss the values c, d and we let them be free variables.

Let us compute torque with respect to the centroid of a tetrahedron to see whether we can set free parameters k, l, c, d to conform on the torque-free condition. Denoting $\mathbf{R}$ the centroid and $\mathbf{T}^1, \mathbf{T}^2$ the respective torques of triangles ABC and ABD, we get

$$
\begin{aligned}
\mathbf{T}^1 &= \mathbf{F}_A^1 \times (\mathbf{A} - \mathbf{R}) + \mathbf{F}_B^1 \times (\mathbf{B} - \mathbf{R}) + \mathbf{F}_C \times (\mathbf{C} - \mathbf{R}) \\
&= -k\mathbf{F}_C \times \mathbf{A} - (1-k)\mathbf{F}_C \times \mathbf{B} \\
&\quad + \mathbf{F}_C \times \mathbf{C} - (\mathbf{F}_A^1 \times \mathbf{R} + \mathbf{F}_B^1 \times \mathbf{R} + \mathbf{F}_C \times \mathbf{R}) \\
&= \mathbf{F}_C \times (-k\mathbf{A} - (1-k)\mathbf{B} + \mathbf{C}) - (\mathbf{F}_A^1 + \mathbf{F}_B^1 + \mathbf{F}_C) \times \mathbf{R}.
\end{aligned}
$$

Similarly we have

$$
\begin{aligned}
\mathbf{T}^2 &= \mathbf{F}_A^2 \times (\mathbf{A} - \mathbf{R}) + \mathbf{F}_B^2 \times (\mathbf{B} - \mathbf{R}) + \mathbf{F}_D \times (\mathbf{D} - \mathbf{R}) \\
&= -l\mathbf{F}_D \times \mathbf{A} - (1-l)\mathbf{F}_D \times \mathbf{B} \\
&\quad + \mathbf{F}_D \times \mathbf{D} - (\mathbf{F}_A^2 \times \mathbf{R} + \mathbf{F}_B^2 \times \mathbf{R} + \mathbf{F}_D \times \mathbf{R}) \\
&= \mathbf{F}_D \times (-l\mathbf{A} - (1-l)\mathbf{B} + \mathbf{D}) - (\mathbf{F}_A^2 + \mathbf{F}_B^2 + \mathbf{F}_D) \times \mathbf{R}.
\end{aligned}
$$

Since we have a force-free condition satisfied for bending forces on each triangle, the last terms in both expressions vanish. Therefore the torques can be computed as

$$
\begin{aligned}
\mathbf{T}^1 &= \mathbf{F}_C \times (-k\mathbf{A} - (1-k)\mathbf{B} + \mathbf{C}) \\
\mathbf{T}^2 &= \mathbf{F}_D \times (-l\mathbf{A} - (1-l)\mathbf{B} + \mathbf{D}).
\end{aligned}
$$

Clearly, the individual torques are non-zero. Indeed, both triangles would start rotating after applying bending forces. They would however rotate in the opposite direction and therefore there is still a chance that $\mathbf{T}^1$ and $\mathbf{T}^2$ cancel out.

Note that $\mathbf{F}_C$ is perpendicular to plane ABC. Properties of a cross-product ensure that $\mathbf{T}^1$ is perpendicular to $\mathbf{F}_C$ and thus $\mathbf{T}^1$ must belong to that plane. Similarly, $\mathbf{F}_D$ belongs to plane ABD. Therefore, the only chance that $\mathbf{T}^1$ cancels out with $\mathbf{T}^2$ is when they are co-linear. Planes ABC and ABD have the only common line AB and, as a consequence, both torques must be multiples of vector $\mathbf{A}-\mathbf{B}$. Choosing another scaling factor m we can eventually write

$$m(\mathbf{A} - \mathbf{B}) = \mathbf{F}_C \times (-k\mathbf{A} - (1 - k)\mathbf{B} + \mathbf{C}) \tag{A.2}$$
$$-m(\mathbf{A} - \mathbf{B}) = \mathbf{F}_D \times (-l\mathbf{A} - (1 - l)\mathbf{B} + \mathbf{D}). \tag{A.3}$$

Now let us do some tedious computations plugging (A.1) into the previous relation

$$m(\mathbf{A} - \mathbf{B}) = c\big[(\mathbf{A} - \mathbf{C}) \times (\mathbf{B} - \mathbf{C})\big] \times (-k\mathbf{A} - (1 - k)\mathbf{B} + \mathbf{C})$$
$$\frac{m}{c}(\mathbf{A} - \mathbf{B}) = (\mathbf{A} \times \mathbf{B} - \mathbf{A} \times \mathbf{C} - \mathbf{C} \times \mathbf{B} + \mathbf{C} \times \mathbf{C})$$
$$\times(-k\mathbf{A} - (1 - k)\mathbf{B} + \mathbf{C}).$$

Since $\mathbf{C} \times \mathbf{C} = 0$ we further get

$$\frac{m}{c}(\mathbf{A} - \mathbf{B}) = -k(\mathbf{A} \times \mathbf{B}) \times \mathbf{A} + k(\mathbf{A} \times \mathbf{C}) \times \mathbf{A} + k(\mathbf{C} \times \mathbf{B}) \times \mathbf{A}$$
$$-(1 - k)(\mathbf{A} \times \mathbf{B}) \times \mathbf{B} + (1 - k)(\mathbf{A} \times \mathbf{C}) \times \mathbf{B}$$
$$+(1 - k)(\mathbf{C} \times \mathbf{B}) \times \mathbf{B}$$
$$+(\mathbf{A} \times \mathbf{B}) \times \mathbf{C} - (\mathbf{A} \times \mathbf{C}) \times \mathbf{C} - (\mathbf{C} \times \mathbf{B}) \times \mathbf{C}.$$

The triple cross-product can be rewritten according to relation

$$(\mathbf{a} \times \mathbf{b}) \times \mathbf{c} = (-\mathbf{b}, \mathbf{c})\mathbf{a} + (\mathbf{a}, \mathbf{c})\mathbf{b},$$

and using this in the previous calculation we end up with

$$\frac{m}{c}(\mathbf{A} - \mathbf{B}) =$$
$$-k[-\mathbf{A}(\mathbf{B}, \mathbf{A}) + \mathbf{B}(\mathbf{A}, \mathbf{A})] + k[-\mathbf{A}(\mathbf{C}, \mathbf{A}) + \mathbf{C}(\mathbf{A}, \mathbf{A})]$$
$$+k[-\mathbf{C}(\mathbf{B}, \mathbf{A}) + \mathbf{B}(\mathbf{C}, \mathbf{A})]$$
$$-(1 - k)[-\mathbf{A}(\mathbf{B}, \mathbf{B}) + \mathbf{B}(\mathbf{A}, \mathbf{B})] + (1 - k)[-\mathbf{A}(\mathbf{C}, \mathbf{B}) + \mathbf{C}(\mathbf{A}, \mathbf{B})]$$
$$+(1 - k)[-\mathbf{C}(\mathbf{B}, \mathbf{B}) + \mathbf{B}(\mathbf{C}, \mathbf{B})]$$
$$+[(-\mathbf{A}(\mathbf{B}, \mathbf{C}) + \mathbf{B}(\mathbf{A}, \mathbf{C})] - [-\mathbf{A}(\mathbf{C}, \mathbf{C}) + \mathbf{C}(\mathbf{A}, \mathbf{C})]$$
$$-[-\mathbf{C}(\mathbf{B}, \mathbf{C}) + \mathbf{B}(\mathbf{C}, \mathbf{C})]$$

$$\frac{m}{c}(\mathbf{A} - \mathbf{B}) =$$
$$k\mathbf{A}(\mathbf{B}, \mathbf{A}) - k\mathbf{B}(\mathbf{A}, \mathbf{A}) - k\mathbf{A}(\mathbf{C}, \mathbf{A}) + k\mathbf{C}(\mathbf{A}, \mathbf{A}) - k\mathbf{C}(\mathbf{B}, \mathbf{A})$$
$$+ k\mathbf{B}(\mathbf{C}, \mathbf{A}) + (1 - k)\mathbf{A}(\mathbf{B}, \mathbf{B}) - (1 - k)\mathbf{B}(\mathbf{A}, \mathbf{B}) - (1 - k)\mathbf{A}(\mathbf{C}, \mathbf{B})$$
$$+ (1 - k)\mathbf{C}(\mathbf{A}, \mathbf{B}) - (1 - k)\mathbf{C}(\mathbf{B}, \mathbf{B}) + (1 - k)\mathbf{B}(\mathbf{C}, \mathbf{B})$$
$$- \mathbf{A}(\mathbf{B}, \mathbf{C}) + \mathbf{B}(\mathbf{A}, \mathbf{C}) + \mathbf{A}(\mathbf{C}, \mathbf{C}) - \mathbf{C}(\mathbf{A}, \mathbf{C}) + \mathbf{C}(\mathbf{B}, \mathbf{C}) - \mathbf{B}(\mathbf{C}, \mathbf{C}).$$

Regrouping the terms with respect to corresponding vectors we get

$$\frac{m}{c}(\mathbf{A} - \mathbf{B}) =$$
$$\left[k\mathbf{A}(\mathbf{B}, \mathbf{A}) - k\mathbf{A}(\mathbf{C}, \mathbf{A}) + (1 - k)\mathbf{A}(\mathbf{B}, \mathbf{B}) \right.$$
$$\left. - (1 - k)\mathbf{A}(\mathbf{C}, \mathbf{B}) - \mathbf{A}(\mathbf{B}, \mathbf{C}) + \mathbf{A}(\mathbf{C}, \mathbf{C}) \right]$$
$$+ \left[- k\mathbf{B}(\mathbf{A}, \mathbf{A}) + k\mathbf{B}(\mathbf{C}, \mathbf{A}) - (1 - k)\mathbf{B}(\mathbf{A}, \mathbf{B}) \right.$$
$$\left. + (1 - k)\mathbf{B}(\mathbf{C}, \mathbf{B}) + \mathbf{B}(\mathbf{A}, \mathbf{C}) - \mathbf{B}(\mathbf{C}, \mathbf{C}) \right]$$
$$+ \left[+ k\mathbf{C}(\mathbf{A}, \mathbf{A})) - k\mathbf{C}(\mathbf{B}, \mathbf{A}) + (1 - k)\mathbf{C}(\mathbf{A}, \mathbf{B}) \right.$$
$$\left. - (1 - k)\mathbf{C}(\mathbf{B}, \mathbf{B}) - \mathbf{C}(\mathbf{A}, \mathbf{C}) + \mathbf{C}(\mathbf{B}, \mathbf{C}) \right. \tag{A.4}$$

$$\frac{m}{c}(\mathbf{A} - \mathbf{B}) = \tag{A.5}$$
$$\mathbf{A}\left[k(\mathbf{B}, \mathbf{A}) - k(\mathbf{C}, \mathbf{A}) + (1 - k)(\mathbf{B}, \mathbf{B}) \right.$$
$$\left. - (1 - k)(\mathbf{C}, \mathbf{B}) - (\mathbf{B}, \mathbf{C}) + (\mathbf{C}, \mathbf{C}) \right]$$
$$+ \mathbf{B}\left[- k(\mathbf{A}, \mathbf{A}) + k(\mathbf{C}, \mathbf{A}) - (1 - k)(\mathbf{A}, \mathbf{B}) \right.$$
$$\left. + (1 - k)(\mathbf{C}, \mathbf{B}) + (\mathbf{A}, \mathbf{C}) - (\mathbf{C}, \mathbf{C}) \right]$$
$$+ \mathbf{C}\left[+ k(\mathbf{A}, \mathbf{A})) - k(\mathbf{B}, \mathbf{A}) + (1 - k)(\mathbf{A}, \mathbf{B}) \right.$$
$$\left. - (1 - k)(\mathbf{B}, \mathbf{B}) - (\mathbf{A}, \mathbf{C}) + (\mathbf{B}, \mathbf{C}) \right].$$

If we want to satisfy the equation with arbitrary choice of $\mathbf{C}$, we need to set the coefficient in front of $\mathbf{C}$ to be zero

$$\begin{aligned} 0 &= k(\mathbf{A}, \mathbf{A})) - k(\mathbf{B}, \mathbf{A}) + (1 - k)(\mathbf{A}, \mathbf{B}) \\ &\quad - (1 - k)(\mathbf{B}, \mathbf{B}) - (\mathbf{A}, \mathbf{C}) + (\mathbf{B}, \mathbf{C}) \\ &= k(\mathbf{A}, \mathbf{A})) - k(\mathbf{B}, \mathbf{A}) + (\mathbf{A}, \mathbf{B}) - k(\mathbf{A}, \mathbf{B}) \\ &\quad - (\mathbf{B}, \mathbf{B}) + k(\mathbf{B}, \mathbf{B}) - (\mathbf{A}, \mathbf{C}) + (\mathbf{B}, \mathbf{C}) \\ &= k\left[(\mathbf{A}, \mathbf{A})) - 2(\mathbf{B}, \mathbf{A}) + (\mathbf{B}, \mathbf{B}) \right] + (\mathbf{A} - \mathbf{B}, \mathbf{B}) - (\mathbf{A} - \mathbf{B}, \mathbf{C}) \\ &= k(\mathbf{A} - \mathbf{B}, \mathbf{A} - \mathbf{B}) + (\mathbf{A} - \mathbf{B}, \mathbf{B} - \mathbf{C}), \end{aligned}$$

which eventually leads to

$$k = \frac{(\mathbf{A} - \mathbf{B}, \mathbf{C} - \mathbf{B})}{(\mathbf{A} - \mathbf{B}, \mathbf{A} - \mathbf{B})}. \tag{A.6}$$

Further, let us put the coefficients in front of $\mathbf{A}$ to be zero

$$
\begin{aligned}
\frac{m}{c} &= k(\mathbf{B}, \mathbf{A}) - k(\mathbf{C}, \mathbf{A}) + (1-k)(\mathbf{B}, \mathbf{B}) \\
&\quad -(1-k)(\mathbf{C}, \mathbf{B}) - (\mathbf{B}, \mathbf{C}) + (\mathbf{C}, \mathbf{C}) \\
&= k(\mathbf{B}-\mathbf{C}, \mathbf{A}) + (\mathbf{B}, \mathbf{B}) - k(\mathbf{B}, \mathbf{B}) - (\mathbf{C}, \mathbf{B}) \\
&\quad + k(\mathbf{C}, \mathbf{B}) - (\mathbf{B}, \mathbf{C}) + (\mathbf{C}, \mathbf{C}) \\
&= k(\mathbf{B}-\mathbf{C}, \mathbf{A}) - k(\mathbf{B}, \mathbf{B}-\mathbf{C}) + (\mathbf{B}-\mathbf{C}, \mathbf{B}-\mathbf{C}) \\
\frac{m}{c} &= k(\mathbf{B}-\mathbf{C}, \mathbf{A}-\mathbf{B}) + (\mathbf{B}-\mathbf{C}, \mathbf{B}-\mathbf{C}). \quad\quad (\text{A.7})
\end{aligned}
$$

Further, let us compute the coefficient in front of $\mathbf{B}$

$$
\begin{aligned}
-\frac{m}{c} &= -k(\mathbf{A}, \mathbf{A}) + k(\mathbf{C}, \mathbf{A}) - (1-k)(\mathbf{A}, \mathbf{B}) \\
&\quad +(1-k)(\mathbf{C}, \mathbf{B}) + (\mathbf{A}, \mathbf{C}) - (\mathbf{C}, \mathbf{C}) \\
&= k(\mathbf{C}-\mathbf{A}, \mathbf{A}) - (\mathbf{A}, \mathbf{B}) + k(\mathbf{A}, \mathbf{B}) + (\mathbf{C}, \mathbf{B}) \\
&\quad -k(\mathbf{C}, \mathbf{B}) + (\mathbf{A}-\mathbf{C}, \mathbf{C}) \\
&= +k(\mathbf{C}-\mathbf{A}, \mathbf{A}) - k(\mathbf{C}-\mathbf{A}, \mathbf{B}) - (\mathbf{A}-\mathbf{C}, \mathbf{B}) + (\mathbf{A}-\mathbf{C}, \mathbf{C}) \\
\frac{m}{c} &= k(\mathbf{C}-\mathbf{A}, \mathbf{A}-\mathbf{B}) - (\mathbf{A}-\mathbf{C}, \mathbf{B}-\mathbf{C}).
\end{aligned}
$$

We can see that we got a different expression for m/c. But we can verify that if we choose such k that (A.6) is satisfied, the previous condition is satisfied automatically. To see this, compute

$$
\begin{aligned}
0 &= \frac{m}{c} - \frac{m}{c} = k(\mathbf{B}-\mathbf{C}, \mathbf{A}-\mathbf{B}) + (\mathbf{B}-\mathbf{C}, \mathbf{B}-\mathbf{C}) \\
&\quad + k(\mathbf{C}-\mathbf{A}, \mathbf{A}-\mathbf{B}) - (\mathbf{A}-\mathbf{C}, \mathbf{B}-\mathbf{C}) \\
&= k(\mathbf{B}-\mathbf{C}+\mathbf{C}-\mathbf{A}, \mathbf{A}-\mathbf{B}) + (\mathbf{B}-\mathbf{C}+\mathbf{C}-\mathbf{A}, \mathbf{B}-\mathbf{C}) \\
&= k(\mathbf{B}-\mathbf{A}, \mathbf{A}-\mathbf{B}) + (\mathbf{B}-\mathbf{A}, \mathbf{B}-\mathbf{C}).
\end{aligned}
$$

Finally, using (A.6) for k we end up with identical zero

$$
\begin{aligned}
&k(\mathbf{B}-\mathbf{A}, \mathbf{A}-\mathbf{B}) + (\mathbf{B}-\mathbf{A}, \mathbf{B}-\mathbf{C}) \\
&= \frac{(\mathbf{A}-\mathbf{B}, \mathbf{C}-\mathbf{B})}{(\mathbf{A}-\mathbf{B}, \mathbf{A}-\mathbf{B})}(\mathbf{B}-\mathbf{A}, \mathbf{A}-\mathbf{B}) + (\mathbf{B}-\mathbf{A}, \mathbf{B}-\mathbf{C}) = 0.
\end{aligned}
$$

To summarise: We analysed (A.2). By computing triple cross-products we came into vectorial equation (A.5). To satisfy this equation we need to have coefficients in front of all three vectors $\mathbf{A}, \mathbf{B}, \mathbf{C}$ to be zero. The question was whether this can be achieved by choosing the right values of k and m/c.

First, we put the coefficient in front of $\mathbf{C}$ in (A.5) to zero. This led us to explicit expression for k given by (A.6). We further put the coefficient in front of $\mathbf{A}$ in (A.5) to zero which led us to explicit expression for m/c given by (A.7). The last step was the verification whether using (A.6) and (A.7) leads to vanishing of the coefficient in front of $\mathbf{B}$. Eventually, it does.

Similar calculations will be done for (A.3)

$$-m(\mathbf{A} - \mathbf{B}) = d\big[(\mathbf{B} - \mathbf{D}) \times (\mathbf{A} - \mathbf{D})\big] \times (-l\mathbf{A} - (1 - l)\mathbf{B} + \mathbf{C})$$

$$\frac{-m}{d}(\mathbf{A} - \mathbf{B}) = [\mathbf{B} \times \mathbf{A} - \mathbf{B} \times \mathbf{D} - \mathbf{D} \times \mathbf{A}] \times (-l\mathbf{A} - (1 - l)\mathbf{B} + \mathbf{D}).$$

We further get

$$
\begin{aligned}
\frac{-m}{d}(\mathbf{A} - \mathbf{B}) = {} & -l(\mathbf{B} \times \mathbf{A}) \times \mathbf{A} + l(\mathbf{B} \times \mathbf{D}) \times \mathbf{A} + l(\mathbf{D} \times \mathbf{A}) \times \mathbf{A} \\
& -(1 - l)(\mathbf{B} \times \mathbf{A}) \times \mathbf{B} + (1 - l)(\mathbf{B} \times \mathbf{D}) \times \mathbf{B} \\
& +(1 - l)(\mathbf{D} \times \mathbf{A}) \times \mathbf{B} \\
& +(\mathbf{B} \times \mathbf{A}) \times \mathbf{D} - (\mathbf{B} \times \mathbf{D}) \times \mathbf{D} - (\mathbf{D} \times \mathbf{A}) \times \mathbf{D},
\end{aligned}
$$

computing the triple cross-product

$$
\begin{aligned}
\frac{-m}{d}(\mathbf{A} - \mathbf{B}) = {} & \\
& -l[-\mathbf{B}(\mathbf{A}, \mathbf{A}) + \mathbf{A}(\mathbf{B}, \mathbf{A})] + l[-\mathbf{B}(\mathbf{D}, \mathbf{A}) + \mathbf{D}(\mathbf{B}, \mathbf{A})] \\
& +l[-\mathbf{D}(\mathbf{A}, \mathbf{A}) + \mathbf{A}(\mathbf{D}, \mathbf{A})] \\
& -(1 - l)[-\mathbf{B}(\mathbf{A}, \mathbf{B}) + \mathbf{A}(\mathbf{B}, \mathbf{B})] + (1 - l)[-\mathbf{B}(\mathbf{D}, \mathbf{B}) + \mathbf{D}(\mathbf{B}, \mathbf{B})] \\
& +(1 - l)[-\mathbf{D}(\mathbf{A}, \mathbf{B}) + \mathbf{A}(\mathbf{D}, \mathbf{B})] \\
& +[(-\mathbf{B}(\mathbf{A}, \mathbf{D}) + \mathbf{A}(\mathbf{B}, \mathbf{D})] - [-\mathbf{B}(\mathbf{D}, \mathbf{D}) + \mathbf{D}(\mathbf{B}, \mathbf{D})] \\
& -[-\mathbf{D}(\mathbf{A}, \mathbf{D}) + \mathbf{A}(\mathbf{D}, \mathbf{D})].
\end{aligned}
$$

Regrouping the terms with respect to corresponding vectors we get

$$
\begin{aligned}
\frac{-m}{d}(\mathbf{A} - \mathbf{B}) = {} & \mathbf{A}\big[-l(\mathbf{B}, \mathbf{A}) + l(\mathbf{D}, \mathbf{A}) - (1 - l)(\mathbf{B}, \mathbf{B}) \\
& \qquad +(1 - l)(\mathbf{D}, \mathbf{B}) + (\mathbf{B}, \mathbf{D}) - (\mathbf{D}, \mathbf{D})\big] \\
& +\mathbf{B}\big[l(\mathbf{A}, \mathbf{A}) - l(\mathbf{D}, \mathbf{A}) + (1 - l)(\mathbf{A}, \mathbf{B}) \\
& \qquad -(1 - l)(\mathbf{D}, \mathbf{B}) - (\mathbf{A}, \mathbf{D}) + (\mathbf{D}, \mathbf{D})\big] \\
& +\mathbf{D}\big[l(\mathbf{B}, \mathbf{A}) - l(\mathbf{A}, \mathbf{A}) + (1 - l)(\mathbf{B}, \mathbf{B}) \\
& \qquad -(1 - l)(\mathbf{A}, \mathbf{B}) - (\mathbf{B}, \mathbf{D}) + (\mathbf{A}, \mathbf{D})\big].
\end{aligned}
$$

Setting the coefficient in front of $\mathbf{D}$ to zero we get

$$
\begin{aligned}
0 = {} & l(\mathbf{B}, \mathbf{A}) - l(\mathbf{A}, \mathbf{A}) + (1 - l)(\mathbf{B}, \mathbf{B}) \\
& -(1 - l)(\mathbf{A}, \mathbf{B}) - (\mathbf{B}, \mathbf{D}) + (\mathbf{A}, \mathbf{D}) \\
= {} & l(\mathbf{B}, \mathbf{A}) - l(\mathbf{A}, \mathbf{A}) + (\mathbf{B}, \mathbf{B}) - l(\mathbf{B}, \mathbf{B}) - (\mathbf{A}, \mathbf{B}) \\
& +l(\mathbf{A}, \mathbf{B}) + (\mathbf{A} - \mathbf{B}, \mathbf{D}) \\
= {} & -l(\mathbf{A} - \mathbf{B}, \mathbf{A} - \mathbf{B}) + (\mathbf{B} - \mathbf{A}, \mathbf{B}) + (\mathbf{A} - \mathbf{B}, \mathbf{D}),
\end{aligned}
$$

which eventually leads to

$$l = \frac{(\mathbf{A} - \mathbf{B}, \mathbf{D} - \mathbf{B})}{(\mathbf{A} - \mathbf{B}, \mathbf{A} - \mathbf{B})}. \tag{A.8}$$

Further, let us put the coefficients in front of $\mathbf{A}$ to be zero

$$
\begin{aligned}
\frac{-m}{d} &= -l(\mathbf{B},\mathbf{A}) + l(\mathbf{D},\mathbf{A}) - (1-l)(\mathbf{B},\mathbf{B}) \\
&\quad +(1-l)(\mathbf{D},\mathbf{B}) + (\mathbf{B},\mathbf{D}) - (\mathbf{D},\mathbf{D}) \\
&= l(\mathbf{D}-\mathbf{B},\mathbf{A}) - (\mathbf{B},\mathbf{B}) + l(\mathbf{B},\mathbf{B}) + (\mathbf{D},\mathbf{B}) \\
&\quad -l(\mathbf{D},\mathbf{B}) + (\mathbf{B}-\mathbf{D},\mathbf{D}) \\
&= l(\mathbf{D}-\mathbf{B},\mathbf{A}) - l(\mathbf{D}-\mathbf{B},\mathbf{B}) - (\mathbf{B}-\mathbf{D},\mathbf{B}) + (\mathbf{B}-\mathbf{D},\mathbf{D}) \\
\frac{-m}{d} &= l(\mathbf{D}-\mathbf{B},\mathbf{A}-\mathbf{B}) + (\mathbf{B}-\mathbf{D},\mathbf{D}-\mathbf{B}). \qquad (A.9)
\end{aligned}
$$

Further, let us compute the coefficient in front of $\mathbf{B}$

$$
\begin{aligned}
\frac{m}{d} &= l(\mathbf{A},\mathbf{A}) - l(\mathbf{D},\mathbf{A}) + (1-l)(\mathbf{A},\mathbf{B}) - (1-l)(\mathbf{D},\mathbf{B}) \\
&\quad -(\mathbf{A},\mathbf{D}) + (\mathbf{D},\mathbf{D}) \\
&= l(\mathbf{A}-\mathbf{D},\mathbf{A}) + (\mathbf{A},\mathbf{B}) - l(\mathbf{A},\mathbf{B}) - (\mathbf{D},\mathbf{B}) \\
&\quad +l(\mathbf{D},\mathbf{B}) + (\mathbf{D}-\mathbf{A},\mathbf{D}) \\
&= l(\mathbf{A}-\mathbf{D},\mathbf{A}) - l(\mathbf{A}-\mathbf{D},\mathbf{B}) - (\mathbf{D}-\mathbf{A},\mathbf{B}) + (\mathbf{D}-\mathbf{A},\mathbf{D}) \\
\frac{m}{d} &= l(\mathbf{A}-\mathbf{D},\mathbf{A}-\mathbf{B}) + (\mathbf{D}-\mathbf{A},\mathbf{D}-\mathbf{B}).
\end{aligned}
$$

Using the expression for $-m/d$ from (A.9), we check whether the expressions cancel out

$$
\begin{aligned}
0 &= \frac{-m}{d} + \frac{m}{d} = l(\mathbf{D}-\mathbf{B},\mathbf{A}-\mathbf{B}) + (\mathbf{B}-\mathbf{D},\mathbf{D}-\mathbf{B}) \\
&\quad +l(\mathbf{A}-\mathbf{D},\mathbf{A}-\mathbf{B}) + (\mathbf{D}-\mathbf{A},\mathbf{D}-\mathbf{B}) \\
&\quad l(\mathbf{D}-\mathbf{B}+\mathbf{A}-\mathbf{D},\mathbf{A}-\mathbf{B}) + (\mathbf{B}-\mathbf{D}+\mathbf{D}-\mathbf{A},\mathbf{D}-\mathbf{B}) \\
&\quad l(\mathbf{A}-\mathbf{B},\mathbf{A}-\mathbf{B}) + (\mathbf{B}-\mathbf{A},\mathbf{D}-\mathbf{B}).
\end{aligned}
$$

Finally, using (A.8) for l we end up with a vanishing coefficient in front of $\mathbf{B}$

$$
\begin{aligned}
&l(\mathbf{A}-\mathbf{B},\mathbf{A}-\mathbf{B}) + (\mathbf{B}-\mathbf{A},\mathbf{D}-\mathbf{B}) \\
&= \frac{(\mathbf{A}-\mathbf{B},\mathbf{D}-\mathbf{B})}{(\mathbf{A}-\mathbf{B},\mathbf{A}-\mathbf{B})}(\mathbf{A}-\mathbf{B},\mathbf{A}-\mathbf{B}) + (\mathbf{B}-\mathbf{A},\mathbf{D}-\mathbf{B}) = 0.
\end{aligned}
$$

To conclude, we list the expressions for $k, l, m/c$ and m/d that lead to force-free and torque-free bending forces

$$
\begin{aligned}
k &= \frac{(\mathbf{A}-\mathbf{B},\mathbf{C}-\mathbf{B})}{(\mathbf{A}-\mathbf{B},\mathbf{A}-\mathbf{B})} \\
\frac{m}{c} &= k(\mathbf{B}-\mathbf{C},\mathbf{A}-\mathbf{B}) + (\mathbf{B}-\mathbf{C},\mathbf{B}-\mathbf{C}) \\
l &= \frac{(\mathbf{A}-\mathbf{B},\mathbf{D}-\mathbf{B})}{(\mathbf{A}-\mathbf{B},\mathbf{A}-\mathbf{B})} \\
\frac{m}{d} &= l(\mathbf{B}-\mathbf{D},\mathbf{A}-\mathbf{B}) + (\mathbf{B}-\mathbf{D},\mathbf{B}-\mathbf{D}). \qquad (A.10)
\end{aligned}
$$

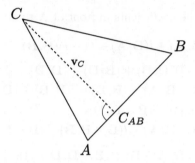

FIGURE A.2: A triangle with altitude $\mathbf{v}_C$ and its foot C_{AB}.

Geometrical insight into the derived bending forces
Let us look in Figure A.2. Here, we have

$$\cos\alpha = \frac{(\mathbf{A} - \mathbf{B}, \mathbf{C} - \mathbf{B})}{|\mathbf{A} - \mathbf{B}||\mathbf{C} - \mathbf{B}|}, \quad |\mathbf{C} - \mathbf{B}|\cos\alpha = \frac{(\mathbf{A} - \mathbf{B}, \mathbf{C} - \mathbf{B})}{|\mathbf{A} - \mathbf{B}|}.$$

Then we have

$$\begin{aligned}
\frac{m}{c} &= k(\mathbf{B} - \mathbf{C}, \mathbf{A} - \mathbf{B}) + (\mathbf{B} - \mathbf{C}, \mathbf{B} - \mathbf{C}) \\
&= -\frac{(\mathbf{A} - \mathbf{B}, \mathbf{C} - \mathbf{B})}{|\mathbf{A} - \mathbf{B}|}\frac{(\mathbf{B} - \mathbf{C}, \mathbf{A} - \mathbf{B})}{|\mathbf{A} - \mathbf{B}|} + |\mathbf{B} - \mathbf{C}|^2 \\
&= -(|\mathbf{C} - \mathbf{B}|\cos\alpha)^2 + |\mathbf{B} - \mathbf{C}|^2 \\
&= |\mathbf{v}_C|^2.
\end{aligned} \tag{A.11}$$

With the same reasoning for triangle ABD we get $m/d = |\mathbf{v}_D|^2$. Since the parameter m is free to choose, the only relation needed to be fulfilled is that

$$\frac{c}{d} = \frac{|\mathbf{v}_D|^2}{|\mathbf{v}_C|^2},$$

which together with relations for k and l ensure that bending is torque-free. Note the definition of c, d in (A.1). Here the cross-products represent double areas of triangles and we can derive that $|\mathbf{F}_C| = cS_{ABC}, |\mathbf{F}_D| = dS_{ABD}$. Putting this together we end up with the following ratio between the forces

$$\frac{|\mathbf{F}_C|}{|\mathbf{F}_D|} = \frac{S_{ABD}}{S_{ABC}},$$

which states that the ratio of magnitudes of bending forces applied to vertices C, D must be inverse to the ratio of the areas of corresponding triangles.

Finally, the bending forces are

$$\mathbf{F}_A = -\beta \frac{mk}{|v_C|^2}\mathbf{N}_C - \beta \frac{ml}{|v_D|^2}\mathbf{N}_D$$

$$\mathbf{F}_B = -\beta \frac{m(1-k)}{|v_C|^2}\mathbf{N}_C - \beta \frac{m(1-l)}{|v_D|^2}\mathbf{N}_D$$

$$\mathbf{F}_C = \beta \frac{m}{|\mathbf{v}_C|^2}\mathbf{N}_C$$

$$\mathbf{F}_D = \beta \frac{m}{|\mathbf{v}_D|^2}\mathbf{N}_D, \qquad (A.12)$$

where $\mathbf{N}_C = (\mathbf{A} - \mathbf{C}) \times (\mathbf{B} - \mathbf{C})$ and $\mathbf{N}_D = (\mathbf{B} - \mathbf{D}) \times (\mathbf{A} - \mathbf{D})$, where $\mathbf{N}_C$ is normal to ABC and $\mathbf{N}_D$ is normal to ABD. Here, the pre-factor $\beta = k_b(\theta - \theta_0)$ is introduced to explicitly show the dependence on the bending coefficient and deviation of the relaxed angle. We discuss the factor m in the next section.

A.2   Comparison to other approaches

In [107], an energy approach is used and the bending forces are derived by differentiating the bending energy of triangles i, j with angle θ_{ij} between them

$$E_{ij}^B = \frac{\kappa_B}{2}(\theta_{ij} - \theta_{ij}^{(0)})^2,$$

with respect to the positions $\mathbf{x}_k$. Therefore

$$\mathbf{F}_k^B = -\kappa_B(\theta_{ij} - \theta_{ij}^{(0)})\frac{\partial \theta_{ij}}{\partial \mathbf{x}_k}.$$

Using the notation from the previous section, the resulting forces in [107] in the points $\mathbf{A}, \mathbf{B}, \mathbf{C}, \mathbf{D}$ are as follows:

$$\mathbf{F}_A^* = \beta \frac{1}{\sqrt{1 - (\mathbf{n}_C, \mathbf{n}_D)^2}}\left[\frac{1}{2S_{ABC}}(\mathbf{C} - \mathbf{B}) \times [\mathbf{n}_D - (\mathbf{n}_C, \mathbf{n}_D)\mathbf{n}_C] \right.$$

$$+ \frac{1}{2S_{ABD}}(\mathbf{B} - \mathbf{D}) \times [\mathbf{n}_C - (\mathbf{n}_C, \mathbf{n}_D)\mathbf{n}_D] \Big]$$

$$\mathbf{F}_B^* = \beta \frac{1}{\sqrt{1 - (\mathbf{n}_C, \mathbf{n}_D)^2}}\left[\frac{1}{2S_{ABC}}(\mathbf{A} - \mathbf{C}) \times [\mathbf{n}_D - (\mathbf{n}_C, \mathbf{n}_D)\mathbf{n}_C] \right.$$

$$+ \frac{1}{2S_{ABD}}(\mathbf{D} - \mathbf{A}) \times [\mathbf{n}_C - (\mathbf{n}_C, \mathbf{n}_D)\mathbf{n}_D] \Big]$$

$$\mathbf{F}_C^* = \beta \frac{1}{\sqrt{1 - (\mathbf{n}_C, \mathbf{n}_D)^2}}\frac{1}{2S_{ABC}}(\mathbf{B} - \mathbf{A}) \times [\mathbf{n}_D - (\mathbf{n}_C, \mathbf{n}_D)\mathbf{n}_C]$$

$$\mathbf{F}_D^* = \beta \frac{1}{\sqrt{1 - (\mathbf{n}_C, \mathbf{n}_D)^2}}\frac{1}{2S_{ABD}}(\mathbf{A} - \mathbf{B}) \times [\mathbf{n}_C - (\mathbf{n}_C, \mathbf{n}_D)\mathbf{n}_D],$$

where $\mathbf{n_C}, \mathbf{n_D}$ are unit normal vectors to triangles ABC, ABD, respectively.

Consider the vector $\mathbf{n_D} - (\mathbf{n_C}, \mathbf{n_D})\mathbf{n_C}$. It is perpendicular to $\mathbf{n_C}$, since

$$\Big([\mathbf{n_D} - (\mathbf{n_C}, \mathbf{n_D})\mathbf{n_C}], \mathbf{n_C}\Big) = (\mathbf{n_D}, \mathbf{n_C}) - (\mathbf{n_C}, \mathbf{n_D})(\mathbf{n_C}, \mathbf{n_C}) = 0.$$

It is also perpendicular to $(\mathbf{A} - \mathbf{B})$, since $\mathbf{n_C} \perp (\mathbf{A} - \mathbf{B})$ and $\mathbf{n_D} \perp (\mathbf{A} - \mathbf{B})$ due to the fact that they are the normal vectors to triangles ABC and ABD, respectively.

This means that the vector $\mathbf{n_D} - (\mathbf{n_C}, \mathbf{n_D})\mathbf{n_C}$ is co-linear with $\mathbf{v}_C$. Its magnitude is

$$
\begin{aligned}
|\mathbf{n_D} - (\mathbf{n_C}, \mathbf{n_D})\mathbf{n_C}|^2 &= |\mathbf{n_D}|^2 - 2(\mathbf{n_C}, \mathbf{n_D}) \cdot (\mathbf{n_C}, \mathbf{n_D}) + |\mathbf{n_C}|^2 (\mathbf{n_C}, \mathbf{n_D})^2 \\
&= 1 - (\mathbf{n_C}, \mathbf{n_D})^2.
\end{aligned}
$$

With this, the force $\mathbf{F}_C^*$ may be re-written as follows (using the fact that the cross-product of two unit vectors that are perpendicular to each other, is also a unit vector):

$$
\begin{aligned}
\mathbf{F}_C^* &= \beta \frac{1}{2S_{ABC}}(\mathbf{B} - \mathbf{A}) \times \frac{\mathbf{v}_C}{|\mathbf{v}_C|} = \\
&= \beta \frac{1}{2S_{ABC}}|\mathbf{B} - \mathbf{A}|\mathbf{n_C} = \\
&= \beta \frac{1}{2S_{ABC}}|\mathbf{B} - \mathbf{A}|\frac{|\mathbf{v}_C|}{|\mathbf{v}_C|}\mathbf{n_C} = \\
&= \beta \frac{S_{ABC}}{S_{ABC}}\frac{1}{|\mathbf{v}_C|}\mathbf{n_C} = \\
&= \frac{\beta}{|\mathbf{v}_C|}\mathbf{n_C}.
\end{aligned}
$$

Similarly

$$\mathbf{F}_D^* = \frac{\beta}{|\mathbf{v}_D|}\mathbf{n_D}.$$

Note that for

$$m = \frac{|\mathbf{v}_C|}{|\mathbf{N}_C|} = \frac{|\mathbf{v}_D|}{|\mathbf{N}_D|} = \frac{1}{|\mathbf{B} - \mathbf{A}|},$$

these $\mathbf{F}_C^*$ and $\mathbf{F}_D^*$ forces are identical to $\mathbf{F}_C$ and $\mathbf{F}_D$, respectively.

Now we do a similar calculation for $\mathbf{F}_A^*$:

$$
\begin{aligned}
\mathbf{F}_A^* &= -\beta \left(\frac{1}{2S_{ABC}}(\mathbf{C} - \mathbf{B}) \times \frac{\mathbf{v}_C}{|\mathbf{v}_C|} + \frac{1}{2S_{ABD}}(\mathbf{B} - \mathbf{D}) \times \frac{\mathbf{v}_D}{|\mathbf{v}_D|} \right) = \\
&= -\beta \left(\frac{1}{2S_{ABC}}|\mathbf{C} - \mathbf{B}| \sin\gamma\mathbf{n_C} + \frac{1}{2S_{ABD}}|\mathbf{B} - \mathbf{D}| \sin\delta\mathbf{n_D} \right) = \\
&= -\beta \left(\frac{|\mathbf{C}_{AB} - \mathbf{B}|}{2S_{ABC}}\mathbf{n_C} + \frac{|\mathbf{D}_{AB} - \mathbf{B}|}{2S_{ABD}}\mathbf{n_D} \right)
\end{aligned}
$$

where $\gamma = \angle C_{AB}CB$ and $\delta = \angle D_{AB}DB$.

And we compare this result to $\mathbf{F}_A$ from (A.12):

$$
\begin{aligned}
\mathbf{F}_A &= -\beta \left(\frac{mk}{v_C^2} \mathbf{N}_C + \frac{ml}{v_D^2} \mathbf{N}_D \right) \\
&= -\beta \left(\frac{mk|\mathbf{B} - \mathbf{A}|}{2S_{ABC}v_C} \mathbf{N}_C + \frac{ml|\mathbf{B} - \mathbf{A}|}{2S_{ABD}v_D} \mathbf{N}_D \right) \\
&= -\beta \left(\frac{k}{2S_{ABC}v_C} \mathbf{N}_C + \frac{l}{2S_{ABD}v_D} \mathbf{N}_D \right) \\
&= -\beta \left(\frac{k}{2S_{ABC}v_C} 2S_{ABC}\mathbf{n}_C + \frac{l}{2S_{ABD}v_D} 2S_{ABD}\mathbf{n}_D \right) \\
&= -\beta \left(\frac{(\mathbf{A} - \mathbf{B}, \mathbf{C} - \mathbf{B})}{|\mathbf{A} - \mathbf{B}|^2 v_C} \mathbf{n}_C + \frac{(\mathbf{A} - \mathbf{B}, \mathbf{D} - \mathbf{B})}{|\mathbf{A} - \mathbf{B}|^2 v_D} \mathbf{n}_D \right) \\
&= -\beta \left(\frac{|\mathbf{A} - \mathbf{B}| \, |\mathbf{C} - \mathbf{B}| \cos \alpha}{|\mathbf{A} - \mathbf{B}|^2 v_C} \mathbf{n}_C + \frac{|\mathbf{A} - \mathbf{B}| \, |\mathbf{D} - \mathbf{B}| \cos \gamma}{|\mathbf{A} - \mathbf{B}|^2 v_D} \mathbf{n}_D \right) \\
&= -\beta \left(\frac{|C_{AB} - \mathbf{B}|}{2S_{ABC}} \mathbf{n}_C + \frac{|D_{AB} - \mathbf{B}|}{2S_{ABD}} \mathbf{n}_D \right),
\end{aligned}
$$

where $\alpha = \angle ABC$ and $\gamma = \angle ABD$. We see that $\mathbf{F}_A^* = \mathbf{F}_A$ and a similar result can be shown for $\mathbf{F}_B^* = \mathbf{F}_B$.

Equivalence of force-based and energy-based definitions of bending modulus

The two approaches: 1. imposing force-free and torque-free conditions on bending forces and 2. differentiating the bending energy, lead to the same, albeit differently written, definition of forces.

Note that the definition of bending forces in [56] is the same up to a multiplicative factor $\beta_b = k_b \sin(\theta - \theta_0)/\sqrt{1 - \cos^2 \theta}$.

Things to ponder

In this approach, if we split the common edge $\mathbf{AB}$ in half and consider the smaller triangles, we get the same bending forces (since they only depend on the altitudes $|v_c|$, $|v_d|$ and the normal vectors). This is counterintuitive because the bending energy on the four smaller triangles would be double the energy on the two larger triangles. What happens if we continue the *division* process? Could it rise even further? Of course, triangulation would not be regular, so this is not something we would do, but is there a flaw in the reasoning? If so, where?

A.3   Computationally friendly expressions

The expressions from the previous section involving $\mathbf{v}_C, \mathbf{v}_D, |\mathbf{C}_{AD} - \mathbf{B}|, |\mathbf{D}_{AB} - \mathbf{B}|$ are not very convenient for computer implementation. To provide expressions involving position vectors $\mathbf{A}, \mathbf{B}, \mathbf{C}$ and $\mathbf{D}$, we need to perform some geometric algebra. From the expression for a double area of a triangle we have

$$|\mathbf{B} - \mathbf{A}||\mathbf{v}_C| = |(\mathbf{A} - \mathbf{B}) \times (\mathbf{B} - \mathbf{C})|, \quad |\mathbf{B} - \mathbf{A}||\mathbf{v}_D| = |(\mathbf{B} - \mathbf{D}) \times (\mathbf{A} - \mathbf{D})|.$$

Further, recall that m from (A.12) is equal to $1/|\mathbf{B} - \mathbf{A}|$ and using relation for k and l from (A.10) in expressions (A.12), we arrive at

$$\mathbf{F}_A = -k_b(\theta - \theta_0)\left(\frac{\mathbf{N}_C}{|\mathbf{N}_C|^2} \frac{(\mathbf{A} - \mathbf{B}, \mathbf{C} - \mathbf{B})}{|\mathbf{B} - \mathbf{A}|} + \frac{\mathbf{N}_D}{|\mathbf{N}_D|^2} \frac{(\mathbf{A} - \mathbf{B}, \mathbf{D} - \mathbf{B})}{|\mathbf{B} - \mathbf{A}|} \right)$$

$$\mathbf{F}_A = -k_b(\theta - \theta_0)\left(\frac{\mathbf{N}_C}{|\mathbf{N}_C|^2} \frac{(\mathbf{A} - \mathbf{B}, \mathbf{A} - \mathbf{D})}{|\mathbf{B} - \mathbf{A}|} + \frac{\mathbf{N}_D}{|\mathbf{N}_D|^2} \frac{(\mathbf{A} - \mathbf{B}, \mathbf{D} - \mathbf{B})}{|\mathbf{B} - \mathbf{A}|} \right)$$

$$\mathbf{F}_C = k_b(\theta - \theta_0)|\mathbf{B} - \mathbf{A}|\frac{\mathbf{N}_C}{|\mathbf{N}_C|^2}$$

$$\mathbf{F}_D = k_b(\theta - \theta_0)|\mathbf{B} - \mathbf{A}|\frac{\mathbf{N}_D}{|\mathbf{N}_D|^2}, \qquad\qquad (A.13)$$

where $\mathbf{N}_C = (\mathbf{A} - \mathbf{C}) \times (\mathbf{B} - \mathbf{C})$ and $\mathbf{N}_D = (\mathbf{B} - \mathbf{D}) \times (\mathbf{A} - \mathbf{D})$.

Appendix B

Comparison of area interactions to other approaches

B.1 Local area interaction

As we have discussed in [102], the following definition of local area is both force- and torque-free:

$$\mathbf{F}_{al}(\mathbf{A}) = -\frac{1}{|\mathbf{t}_A|^2 + |\mathbf{t}_B|^2 + |\mathbf{t}_C|^2} k_{al} \Delta S_{ABC} \mathbf{t}_A,$$

where $\mathbf{T}$ is the centroid of triangle ABC and $\mathbf{t}_A = \mathbf{T} - \mathbf{A}$, with analogous expressions for vertices $\mathbf{B}$ and $\mathbf{C}$.

Let us compare this to the approach in [56], where

$$\mathbf{F}_{al}(\mathbf{A}) = \alpha \mathbf{N} \times (\mathbf{C} - \mathbf{B}).$$

Here $\mathbf{N} = (\mathbf{B} - \mathbf{A}) \times (\mathbf{C} - \mathbf{A})$ is the outer normal vector of the triangle ABC. The cross-product gives a vector which lies in the triangle plane and is perpendicular to the edge BC. There are two different coefficients α, since this type of force is used at two different places.

In the first case $\alpha = qC_q/4S_{ABC}^q$ and this is for the area contribution, which is part of the in-plane modulus. Since in [56] (page 40) the spring potentials are purely attractive (FENE or WLC), they are also responsible for area compression. This work also provides calculation of exponent q and constant C_q that enter the definition of α. This modulus is doing just area expansion. For springs that also have repulsive potential (such as harmonic, or ours), the C_q is set to zero, which means no contribution.

In the second case $\alpha = -k_{al} \Delta S_{ABC}/(4S_{ABC}^0 S_{ABC})$. Since $|\mathbf{N} \times (\mathbf{C} - \mathbf{B})| =$

$2S_{ABC}|\mathbf{C} - \mathbf{B}|$, we get

$$
\begin{aligned}
\mathbf{F}_{al}(\mathbf{A}) &= \alpha \mathbf{N} \times (\mathbf{C} - \mathbf{B}) \\
&= -k_{al} \frac{\Delta S_{ABC} 2 S_{ABC} |\mathbf{C} - \mathbf{B}| \mathbf{v}}{4 S_{ABC}^0 S_{ABC}}, \\
&= -\frac{|\mathbf{C} - \mathbf{B}|}{2 S_{ABC}^0} k_{al} \Delta S_{ABC} \mathbf{v},
\end{aligned}
$$

where $\mathbf{v}$ is the unit vector in the direction of the *altitude*.

DPD local area force effects on regularity of triangulation
In any given triangle, this area force will have the largest contribution in the vertex opposite the longest triangle side and the smallest in the vertex that lies opposite the shortest triangle side. For obtuse triangles the expanding area force tends to regularize the triangulation, however, the compression area force will make the triangles even more obtuse, which might lead to numerical problems when dealing with large deformations.

In [107], the local area force is incorporated into the strain force, so we cannot make a direct comparison.

B.2   Global area interaction

The global area force is defined as

$$
\mathbf{F}_{ag}(A) = -k_{ag} \frac{S^c - S_0^c}{|\mathbf{t}_A|^2 + |\mathbf{t}_B|^2 + |\mathbf{t}_C|^2} \mathbf{t}_A,
$$

the same way as the local force, with the difference that the whole cell surface, S^c and S_0^c, is taken into account.

Both [107] and [56] derive global area force as

$$
\mathbf{F}_{ag}^*(A) = -k_{ag} \frac{S^c - S_0^c}{2 S_0^c} \mathbf{N} \times (\mathbf{C} - \mathbf{B}),
$$

which similarly to the derivation in the previous section acts in the direction of altitude in the triangle ABC. This is similar for vertices B and C.

Appendix C

Force- and torque-free volume modulus

C.1 Global volume interaction

Let us analyse whether our implementation is force free. The relation (3.7) can be rewritten using the fact that

$$\mathbf{n}_{ABC} = \frac{(\mathbf{B} - \mathbf{A}) \times (\mathbf{C} - \mathbf{A})}{2S_{ABC}}.$$

In what follows, we replace notation for points A, B, C with $X_1 X_2 X_3$ for further compatibility with summations over a general number of points larger than three. The volume force corresponding to triangle $X_1 X_2 X_3$ applied to mesh point X_1 can be written as

$$\mathbf{F}_1 = -k_v \frac{V - V_0}{V_0} S_{X_1 X_2 X_3} \frac{\mathbf{n}_{X_1 X_2 X_3}}{3} = -k_V \frac{V - V_0}{V_0} \frac{1}{6} (\mathbf{X}_2 - \mathbf{X}_1) \times (\mathbf{X}_3 - \mathbf{X}_1). \tag{C.1}$$

The sum over one triangle gives us

$$
\begin{aligned}
\mathbf{F}_1 + \mathbf{F}_2 + \mathbf{F}_3 &= \beta \big[(\mathbf{X}_2 - \mathbf{X}_1) \times (\mathbf{X}_3 - \mathbf{X}_1) \\
&\quad + (\mathbf{X}_3 - \mathbf{X}_2) \times (\mathbf{X}_1 - \mathbf{X}_2) \\
&\quad + (\mathbf{X}_1 - \mathbf{X}_3) \times (\mathbf{X}_2 - \mathbf{X}_3) \big] \\
&= 3\beta \big[\mathbf{X}_2 \times \mathbf{X}_3 + \mathbf{X}_3 \times \mathbf{X}_1 + \mathbf{X}_1 \times \mathbf{X}_2 \big],
\end{aligned}
$$

where $\beta = -k_V \frac{V - V_0}{V_0} \frac{1}{6}$.

Let us now consider the total volume force that can be obtained by summation of such contributions over all mesh triangles. Consider one specific edge $X_2 X_3$ from Figure C.1. In the overall sum above, the cross-product $\mathbf{X}_2 \times \mathbf{X}_3$ will be present once due to triangle $X_1 X_2 X_3$ and cross-product $\mathbf{X}_3 \times \mathbf{X}_2$ will also be present once, this time from triangle $X_3 X_2 X_4$. Note, that the order

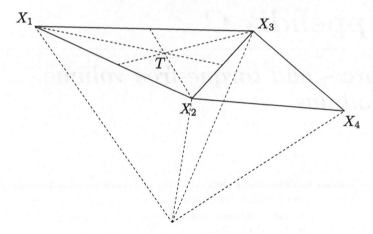

FIGURE C.1: Two adjacent triangles.

of vectors in cross-products is interchanged, and this was due to the proper orientation of the triangles such that normal vectors need to point out of the mesh. These two cross-products cancel out. Since this can be said for each edge of the mesh, the total net force vanishes and volume contribution is force-free.

Computation of torque is more complicated. The torque of the overall volume contribution with respect to centroid located at the origin is equal to the sum of torques of individual mesh points

$$\mathbf{T} = \sum_i \mathbf{X}_i \times \mathbf{F}_i^*,$$

where $\mathbf{F}_i^*$ is the resultant of the forces applied to $\mathbf{X}_i$. Let us compute this contribution for an arbitrary mesh point. Without loss on generality, denote this mesh point by $\mathbf{X}_0$ and the surrounding meshpoints from adjacent triangles will be denoted by $\mathbf{X}_1, \mathbf{X}_2, \ldots, \mathbf{X}_k$ as in Figure C.2. Typically, k equals to 5, 6 or 7 in triangular meshes with non-degenerate triangles. Such meshes have the best numerical properties.

The resultant force $\mathbf{F}_i^*$ is then computed as

$$\mathbf{F}_i^* = \beta \sum_{i=1}^{k} (\mathbf{X}_i - \mathbf{X}_0) \times (\mathbf{X}_{i+1} - \mathbf{X}_0),$$

where $\beta = -k_V \frac{V - V_0}{V_0} \frac{1}{6}$ and we put $\mathbf{X}_{k+1} \equiv \mathbf{X}_1$. The previous expression can be reduced to

$$\mathbf{F}_i^* = \beta \sum_{i=1}^{k} (\mathbf{X}_i \times \mathbf{X}_{i+1}), \qquad (\text{C.2})$$

which leads to the following contribution of mesh point $\mathbf{X}_0$ in total torque

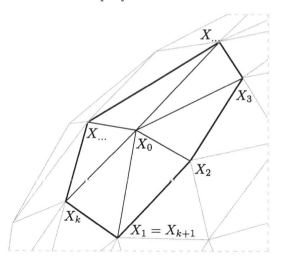

FIGURE C.2: Part of the mesh.

computation:

$$\mathbf{T}_0 = \beta \mathbf{X}_0 \times \sum_{i=1}^{k} (\mathbf{X}_i \times \mathbf{X}_{i+1}).$$

Now we rearrange the terms in total torque computation such that each of k expressions is linked to the corresponding triangle. We do this not only for mesh point $\mathbf{X}_0$ but for all points in the mesh. This way, each triangle gets one term from each of its vertices. For triangle $\mathbf{X}_0\mathbf{X}_1\mathbf{X}_2$ in particluar, we get the following sum:

$$\beta \left[\mathbf{X}_0 \times (\mathbf{X}_1 \times \mathbf{X}_2) + \mathbf{X}_1 \times (\mathbf{X}_2 \times \mathbf{X}_0) + \mathbf{X}_2 \times (\mathbf{X}_0 \times \mathbf{X}_1) \right],$$

which eventually cancels out. Performing this action for each triangle, we end up with vanishing torque with respect to the centroid of the net mesh.

C.2 Comparison to other approaches

In [107] the volume conservation is mediated via a volume energy given by

$$E_V = \frac{k_V}{2} \frac{(V - V_0)^2}{V_0}. \tag{C.3}$$

The corresponding volume forces are derived by differentiation of the energy with respect to spatial position

$$\mathbf{F}_V = -\frac{\partial E_V(\mathbf{X})}{\partial \mathbf{X}} = -k_V \frac{V - V_0}{V_0} \frac{\partial V(\mathbf{X})}{\partial \mathbf{X}}, \tag{C.4}$$

where volume can be expressed as

$$V = \frac{1}{6}(\mathbf{X}_3 \times \mathbf{X}_2, \mathbf{X}_1),$$

leading to

$$\frac{\partial V(\mathbf{X})}{\partial \mathbf{X}_1} = \frac{1}{6}(\mathbf{X}_2 \times \mathbf{X}_3), \tag{C.5}$$

where X_1, X_2, X_3 are points of one triangle from the mesh.

This approach is identical to that from [56]. Here, the resulting forces are written in a different way:

$$\frac{\partial V(\mathbf{X})}{\partial \mathbf{X}_1} = \frac{1}{6}\left(\frac{\mathbf{N}_1}{3} + \mathbf{C} \times (\mathbf{X}_3 - \mathbf{X}_2)\right), \tag{C.6}$$

where $\mathbf{N}_1$ is a vector perpendicular to $\mathbf{X}_1\mathbf{X}_2\mathbf{X}_3$ defined as $\mathbf{N}_1 = (\mathbf{X}_2 - \mathbf{X}_1) \times (\mathbf{X}_3 - \mathbf{X}_1)$ and $\mathbf{C}$ is the centroid of triangle $\mathbf{X}_1\mathbf{X}_2\mathbf{X}_3$. Using the expression for a centroid, a simple calculation reveals the identity between two approaches:

$$\frac{1}{6}\left(\frac{\mathbf{N}_1}{3} + \mathbf{C} \times (\mathbf{X}_3 - \mathbf{X}_2)\right)$$

$$= \frac{1}{6}\left(\frac{(\mathbf{X}_2 - \mathbf{X}_1) \times (\mathbf{X}_3 - \mathbf{X}_1)}{3} + \frac{\mathbf{X}_1 + \mathbf{X}_2 + \mathbf{X}_3}{3} \times (\mathbf{X}_3 - \mathbf{X}_2)\right)$$

$$= \frac{1}{6}\left(\frac{(\mathbf{X}_2 \times \mathbf{X}_3 - \mathbf{X}_2 \times \mathbf{X}_1 - \mathbf{X}_1 \times \mathbf{X}_3}{3}\right.$$

$$\left. + \frac{\mathbf{X}_1 \times \mathbf{X}_3 + \mathbf{X}_2 \times \mathbf{X}_3 - \mathbf{X}_1 \times \mathbf{X}_2 - \mathbf{X}_3 \times \mathbf{X}_2}{3}\right)$$

$$= \frac{1}{6}\frac{3(\mathbf{X}_2 \times \mathbf{X}_3)}{3} = \frac{1}{6}(\mathbf{X}_2 \times \mathbf{X}_3).$$

It is quite easy to verify that this implementation is force-free. Total net force in a mesh is equal to

$$\sum_{ijk}(\mathbf{X}_i \times \mathbf{X}_j + \mathbf{X}_j \times \mathbf{X}_k + \mathbf{X}_k \times \mathbf{X}_i),$$

where the summing is done over all triples ijk such that triangle $\mathbf{X}_i\mathbf{X}_j\mathbf{X}_k$ belongs to the mesh and is properly oriented. Similarly as before, consider one specific edge X_2X_3 as in Figure C.1. In the overall sum above, the cross-product $\mathbf{X}_2 \times \mathbf{X}_3$ will be present once due to triangle $X_1X_2X_3$ and cross-product $\mathbf{X}_3 \times \mathbf{X}_2$ will also be present once, cancelling each other out. This can be said for each edge of the mesh and thus the total net force is zero.

Regarding the torque, the computation for one triangle $\mathbf{X}_1\mathbf{X}_2\mathbf{X}_3$ reveals that

$$
\begin{aligned}
\mathbf{T}_{123} &= \mathbf{X}_1 \times (\mathbf{X}_2 \times \mathbf{X}_3) + \mathbf{X}_2 \times (\mathbf{X}_3 \times \mathbf{X}_1) + \mathbf{X}_3 \times (\mathbf{X}_1 \times \mathbf{X}_2) \\
&= (\mathbf{X}_1, \mathbf{X}_3)\mathbf{X}_2 - (\mathbf{X}_1, \mathbf{X}_2)\mathbf{X}_3 + (\mathbf{X}_2, \mathbf{X}_1)\mathbf{X}_3 \\
&\quad -(\mathbf{X}_2, \mathbf{X}_3)\mathbf{X}_1 + (\mathbf{X}_3, \mathbf{X}_2)\mathbf{X}_1) - (\mathbf{X}_3, \mathbf{X}_1)\mathbf{X}_2 = 0.
\end{aligned}
$$

Here, we used the assumption that the center of mass of the mesh is located at the origin. Summing the torque over all triangles we get zero torque of the volume force with respect to centroid of the mesh. Since the net force is zero, the torque vanished with respect to an arbitrary point in space, too.

C.3 In-plane or out-of-plane volume forces

The Occam's razor principle states that *simple is good* or more specific *Among competing hypotheses, the one with the fewest assumptions should be selected.* Following this principle, one could say that the approach for volume modulus based on the volume energy (C.3) is the winner when competing in the *best volume implementation* race. The expression for the energy is simple, logical and straightforward. The expressions for the volume forces that are derived by differentiation of the energy with respect to position are also quite simple, so there is no need for digging deeper and looking for another approach.

Still, we should not condemn the first-forces-then-energy approach. By (3.7) we define forces for volume modulus that have one significant advantage over the other approach: The forces are out-of-plane.

Indeed, in (C.6) we see that the forces are composed of two components. An out-of-plane component represented by $\mathbf{N}_1$ and a component $\mathbf{C} \times (\mathbf{X}_3 - \mathbf{X}_2)$. The latter vector is definitely not perpendicular to plane $\mathbf{X}_1\mathbf{X}_2\mathbf{X}_3$ and even for regular meshes, where vector C is perpendicular to plane $\mathbf{X}_1\mathbf{X}_2\mathbf{X}_3$, the second component is in-line.

In the view of competing moduli, presented in Section 3.4.3, the decision of what implementation of volume modulus is more advantageous is not decided yet. The answer will be given in Section C.4.

C.4 Search for the volume energy

Let us find out whether it is possible to find an energy function such that its derivative gives the force expressions (C.1). From the previous section we know that if we differentiate the energy given by (C.4), we end up with (C.5) which is equivalent to (C.6). Since our forces have the form very similar to the latter, the first attempt is to modify V to some other function $U = U(\mathbf{X}_1) : R^3 \to R$ such that

$$\frac{\partial U(\mathbf{X}_1)}{\partial \mathbf{X}_1} = \frac{1}{6}\mathbf{N}_1 = \mathbf{X}_3 \times \mathbf{X}_2 + \mathbf{X}_1 \times (\mathbf{X}_3 - \mathbf{X}_2). \tag{C.7}$$

If we succeed in finding U we will have the energy equal

$$E_V = \frac{k_V}{2}\frac{(U - V_0)^2}{V_0}$$

Unfortunately, it is not possible to find such U. By setting the general form $U(\mathbf{X}_1)$ as a quadratic function of components of $\mathbf{X}_1$, we end up with the condition that $\mathbf{X}_2 = \mathbf{X}_3$. This also has a geometric reason. If we first subtract from U the V denoting $\Delta(\mathbf{X}_1) = U - V$ we are looking for Δ such that

$$\frac{\partial \Delta(\mathbf{X}_1)}{\partial \mathbf{X}_1} = \mathbf{X}_1 \times (\mathbf{X}_3 - \mathbf{X}_2).$$

This however means that we are looking for a function with its gradient perpendicular to the vector field $\mathbf{X}_1$. Recall the following property of a gradient: Gradient $\Delta(\mathbf{X}_1)$ is always perpendicular to the tangent plane to the level curve $\Delta(\mathbf{X}_1) = const$. Putting this together with the fact that the gradient must be perpendicular to $\mathbf{X}_1$ we end up with zero gradient.

To find the energy for (C.1) we need to be careful. We have a global expression V in that relation. We can split V as the sum of individual volumes V_j being the volumes of tetrahedra having one side the face of a mesh and the fourth vertex the centroid of the mesh. But when computing $\partial E/\partial \mathbf{X}_1$ we have to be aware that not only one of the volumes V_j is dependent on $\mathbf{X}_1$, but several. These volumes form a *cap* around the vertex $\mathbf{X}_1$. So we need to realise that in the expression

$$\frac{\partial U(\mathbf{X}_1)}{\partial \mathbf{X}_1} = -k_V\frac{V(\mathbf{X}_1) - V_0}{V_0}\frac{1}{6}(\mathbf{X}_3 \times \mathbf{X}_2 + \mathbf{X}_1 \times (\mathbf{X}_3 - \mathbf{X}_2)), \tag{C.8}$$

the term $V(\mathbf{X}_1)$ can be expressed as a sum of several individual volumes from a cap. Therefore, we need to look at this expression not at each individual volume separately, but we need to sum up forces in each vertex for all individual volumes from the cap, and only afterwards, look for the energy U. Saying that, we reformulate the problem.

We search for U such that for each vertex (we use the representative index 1) we have

$$\frac{\partial U(\mathbf{X}_1)}{\partial \mathbf{X}_1} = -k_V\frac{V_{cap}(\mathbf{X}_1) - V_0}{V_0}\frac{1}{6}(\mathbf{X}_3 \times \mathbf{X}_2 + \mathbf{X}_1 \times (\mathbf{X}_3 - \mathbf{X}_2)), \tag{C.9}$$

where

$$V_{cap} = \sum_{j \in cap} V_j.$$

Now recall (C.2). Here we see that resultant force in a vertex $\mathbf{X}_1$ may be written as the sum of cross-products from vectors around $\mathbf{X}_1$ belonging to the *cap*, but a closer look reveals that the resultant force in $\mathbf{X}_1$ in our approach is identical to the resultant force in $\mathbf{X}_1$ in the IBM [107] and DPD [56] approaches.

To conclude:

DPD, IBM and IB-DC comparison

In a search for the energy in the IB-DC approach, we arrived at the same expression for the energy as in IBM and DPD approaches and we have verified that the resultant volume force in our approach is identical to the resultant force in the IBM and DPD approaches. More specifically, although we have different explicit expressions for volume forces in our approach and IBM and DPD approaches, and we pointed out that our approach is out-of-plane and the IBM and DPD approaches are not, in global, when looking at the resultant force per each vertex, the approaches are equivalent, yielding the same volume force per each vertex, when volume forces from all mesh points are summed up.

Appendix D

Calculus of spring network deformations

D.1   Shear modulus

When using regular triangular spring networks, one would like to relate the spring stiffness constants to the physical membrane constants defining the shear modulus μ_0 and the area compression/extension modulus K. Adopting the notation from [40] we have the situation depicted in Figure 4.5. Vectors $\mathbf{a}$ and $\mathbf{b}$ define the geometry of the network and denoting $\mathbf{c} = \mathbf{b} - \mathbf{a} = [b_x - a_x, b_y - a_y]$ we have the following relations:

$$a = |\mathbf{a}| = \sqrt{a_x^2 + a_y^2}, \quad b = |\mathbf{b}| = \sqrt{b_x^2 + b_y^2},$$
$$c = |\mathbf{c}| = \sqrt{(b_x - a_x)^2 + (b_y - a_y)^2}$$

$$(\text{D.1})$$

For areas of the triangles we have

$$A_0 = A_1 = A_2 = A = \frac{1}{2}|\mathbf{a} \times \mathbf{b}| = \frac{1}{2}|a_x b_y - a_y b_x|.$$

Consider the reference lattice in equilibrium, so that the triangles in Figure 4.5 are equilateral with the side length equal to l_0. The vectors in equilibrium are denoted with superscript 0. Then the coordinates of the vectors are as follows:

$$\mathbf{a}^0 = l_0 \left[\frac{\sqrt{3}}{2}, \frac{1}{2}\right], \quad \mathbf{b}^0 = l_0[0, 1], \quad \mathbf{c}^0 = l_0\left[-\frac{\sqrt{3}}{2}, \frac{1}{2}\right].$$

Let us apply an incremental engineering shear strain on this regular triangular lattice given by matrix

$$J = \begin{bmatrix} 1 & \gamma/2 \\ \gamma/2 & 1 \end{bmatrix}, \quad \mathbf{r} = \mathbf{r}^0 J.$$

For small values of $\gamma > 0$, the corresponding deformation involves pure shear. Then we have the following coordinates for the transformed vectors:

$$\mathbf{a} = l_0\left[\frac{\sqrt{3}}{2} + \frac{\gamma}{4}, \frac{1}{2} + \frac{\sqrt{3}\gamma}{4}\right], \quad \mathbf{b} = l_0\left[\frac{\gamma}{2}, 1\right], \quad \mathbf{c} = l_0\left[-\frac{\sqrt{3}}{2} + \frac{\gamma}{4}, \frac{1}{2} - \frac{\sqrt{3}\gamma}{4}\right].$$

Note, that after applying the engineering strain the vectors around the central point are transformed in such a way that all six triangles stay identical up to the rotation.

Let us precompute several quantities. For the area A we get

$$A = \frac{1}{2}l_0^2\left[(\frac{\sqrt{3}}{2} + \frac{\gamma}{4}) - (\frac{1}{2} + \frac{\sqrt{3}\gamma}{4})\frac{\gamma}{2}\right] = \frac{1}{2}l_0^2\left[\frac{\sqrt{3}}{2} + \frac{\sqrt{3}\gamma^2}{8}\right] = \frac{\sqrt{3}l_0^2}{4} + o(\gamma^2).$$

For lengths a, b, c we have

$$a = |\mathbf{a}| = l_0\sqrt{(\frac{\sqrt{3}}{2} + \frac{\gamma}{4})^2 + (\frac{1}{2} + \frac{\sqrt{3}\gamma}{4})^2} = l_0\sqrt{1 + \frac{\sqrt{3}}{2}\gamma + \frac{\gamma^2}{4}}.$$

Using the Taylor expansion of function $a(\gamma)$ we get

$$a = l_0(1 + \frac{\sqrt{3}}{4}\gamma) + o(\gamma^2).$$

For b we get a simpler expression

$$b = |\mathbf{b}| = l_0\sqrt{1 + \gamma^2} = l_0 + o(\gamma^2).$$

Finally for c we obtain

$$c = |\mathbf{c}| = l_0\sqrt{(-\frac{\sqrt{3}}{2} + \frac{\gamma}{4})^2 + (\frac{1}{2} - \frac{\sqrt{3}\gamma}{4})^2} = l_0\sqrt{1 - \frac{\sqrt{3}}{2}\gamma + \frac{\gamma^2}{4}}.$$

Using the Taylor expansion of function $c(\gamma)$ we get

$$c = l_0(1 - \frac{\sqrt{3}}{4}\gamma) + o(\gamma^2).$$

The expressions for magnitudes of stretching forces along the respective edges read as

$$\begin{aligned}
F_a &= k_s(a - a^0) = k_s(l_0(1 + \frac{\sqrt{3}}{4}\gamma) + o(\gamma^2) - l_0) = k_s l_0\gamma\frac{\sqrt{3}}{4} + o(\gamma^2) \\
F_b &= k_s(b - b^0) = k_s(l_0 + o(\gamma^2) - l_0) = o(\gamma^2) \\
F_c &= k_s(c - c^0) = k_s(l_0(1 - \frac{\sqrt{3}}{4}\gamma) + o(\gamma^2) - l_0) = -k_s l_0\gamma\frac{\sqrt{3}}{4} + o(\gamma^2).
\end{aligned}$$

D.2 Area expansion modulus

Biological membranes are probed to get the area expansion modulus. This means that a piece of membrane is being stretched in both directions and the membrane's resistance to the forces is quantified by the area expansion modulus K. In (4.2) we derived the following expression for the area expansion modulus:

$$K = A_0 \left. \frac{dP}{dA} \right|_{A=A_0} \qquad (D.2)$$

where A is the current area of the stretched membrane, A_0 is the relaxed area and P is the diagonal membrane pressure given by

$$P = -\frac{1}{2}(\sigma_{xx} + \sigma_{yy}). \qquad (D.3)$$

Our aim is now to introduce deformation of a regular triangular network corresponding to the expansion. Let us consider the parametrisation of the this network as depicted in Figure 4.6. Parameter x gives us for $x = 1$ the relaxed state, $x > 1$ gives uniform expansion. The individual terms as function of x that are necessary for computation of σ_{xx} and σ_{yy} are the following:

$$a = b = c = xl_0, \quad a_x = \frac{\sqrt{3}}{2}xl_0, \quad a_y = \frac{1}{2}xl_0, \quad b_x = 0, \quad b_y = xl_0,$$

$$c_x = -\frac{\sqrt{3}}{2}xl_0, \quad c_y = \frac{1}{2}xl_0, \quad t_a = |\mathbf{t}_a|, t_b = |\mathbf{t}_b|, t_c = |\mathbf{t}_c|,$$

$$t_a^2 = t_b^2 = t_c^2 = \frac{1}{3}x^2 l_0^2, \quad t_a^2 + t_b^2 + t_c^2 = x^2 l_0^2,$$

$$S_\triangle = \frac{\sqrt{3}}{4}x^2 l_0^2, \quad \Delta S_\triangle = \frac{\sqrt{3}}{4}(x^2 - 1)l_0^2. \qquad (D.4)$$

For two-body forces induced by linear springs with stiffness k_s and relaxed length l_0 we have the following magnitudes of forces:

$$F_a = F_b = F_c = k_s(x - 1)l_0$$

Since we have area expansion mode, the forces for area preservation modulus must be included. For completeness, we need to take into account both local and global area forces. Our implementation of the local area modulus described in Section 3.2 uses the following expression for forces:

$$\mathbf{F}_{AT} = k_{al}\Delta S_\triangle \frac{\mathbf{t}_a}{t_a^2 + t_b^2 + t_c^2}. \qquad (D.5)$$

For global area forces we use (3.9) stating

$$\mathbf{F}_{AT}^g = k_{ag} \frac{S_\triangle}{S_0^c} \Delta S^c \frac{\mathbf{t}_a}{t_a^2 + t_b^2 + t_c^2},$$

where S_0^c is the total surface of relaxed cell and ΔS^c is the deviation of total surface from S_0^c.

If we decompose $\mathbf{F}_{AT}$ into sum of forces acting along the edges AC and AB we get the following:

$$\mathbf{F}_{ACB} = k_{al} \frac{\mathbf{C} - \mathbf{A}}{3} \frac{\Delta S_\triangle}{t_a^2 + t_b^2 + t_c^2}, \quad \mathbf{F}_{ABC} = k_{al} \frac{\mathbf{B} - \mathbf{A}}{3} \frac{\Delta S_\triangle}{t_a^2 + t_b^2 + t_c^2}.$$

For global area contribution we get

$$\mathbf{F}_{ACB}^g = k_{ag} \frac{\mathbf{C} - \mathbf{A}}{3} \frac{\Delta S^c}{t_a^2 + t_b^2 + t_c^2} \frac{S_\triangle}{S_0^c}, \quad \mathbf{F}_{ABC}^g = k_{ag} \frac{\mathbf{B} - \mathbf{A}}{3} \frac{\Delta S^c}{t_a^2 + t_b^2 + t_c^2} \frac{S_\triangle}{S_0^c}.$$

These expressions allow us to evaluate the magnitude of force F_{012} from the expression for the virial in case of three-body forces (4.9):

$$F_{ABC} = F_{ACB} = F_{012} = F_{021} = k_{al} \frac{x l_0}{3} \frac{\frac{\sqrt{3}}{4}(x^2 - 1)l_0^2}{x^2 l_0^2} = k_{al} l_0 \frac{\sqrt{3}}{12} \frac{x^2 - 1}{x}.$$

To derive formulas for global area with N_t triangles in a mesh, note that

$$\Delta S^c = N_t \Delta S_\triangle \quad \text{and} \quad S_0^c = N_t S^0,$$

which leads to

$$\Delta S^c \frac{S_\triangle}{S_0^c} = N_t \Delta S_\triangle \frac{S_\triangle}{N_t S^0} = \Delta S_\triangle \frac{S_\triangle}{S^0} = \Delta S_\triangle x^2.$$

Thus the number of triangles N_t cancels out and we have

$$F_{012}^g = F_{021}^g = k_{ag} l_0 \frac{\sqrt{3}}{12} \frac{x^2 - 1}{x} x^2.$$

Now we are going to evaluate two-body contributions using (4.8), but instead of computing shear stress τ_{xy} we evaluate normal stresses σ_{xx}, σ_{yy} with corresponding changes in (4.8) regarding components a_x and a_y where necessary:

$$\sigma_{xx} = \frac{1}{2S_\triangle}\left[\frac{F_a}{a}a_x a_x + \frac{F_b}{b}b_x b_x + \frac{F_c}{c}c_x c_x\right]$$

$$= \frac{1}{2\frac{\sqrt{3}}{4}x^2 l_0^2}\left[\frac{k_s(x-1)l_0}{xl_0}(\frac{\sqrt{3}}{2}xl_0)^2 + \frac{k_s(x-1)l_0}{xl_0}(-\frac{\sqrt{3}}{2}xl_0)^2\right]$$

$$= \frac{2}{\sqrt{3}x^2 l_0^2}\left[2\frac{k_s(x-1)}{x}\frac{3}{4}x^2 l_0^2\right]$$

$$= k_s\sqrt{3}\frac{x-1}{x}$$

$$\sigma_{yy} = \frac{1}{2S_\triangle}\left[\frac{F_a}{a}a_y a_y + \frac{F_b}{b}b_y b_y + \frac{F_c}{c}c_y c_y\right]$$

$$= \frac{1}{2\frac{\sqrt{3}}{4}x^2 l_0^2}\left[\frac{k_s(x-1)l_0}{xl_0}(\frac{1}{2}xl_0)^2 + \frac{k_s(x-1)l_0}{xl_0}(xl_0)^2\right.$$

$$\left.+\frac{k_s(x-1)l_0}{xl_0}(\frac{1}{2}xl_0)^2\right]$$

$$= \frac{1}{2\frac{\sqrt{3}}{4}x^2 l_0^2}\frac{k_s(x-1)l_0}{xl_0}\left[(\frac{1}{2}xl_0)^2 + (xl_0)^2 + (\frac{1}{2}xl_0)^2\right]$$

$$= \frac{2}{\sqrt{3}x^2 l_0^2}\frac{k_s(x-1)}{x}\left[\frac{3}{2}x^2 l_0^2\right]$$

$$= k_s\sqrt{3}\frac{x-1}{x}. \tag{D.6}$$

Further, we continue with three-body interactions involving local area force using (4.9) but again instead of computing shear stress τ_{xy}, we evaluate normal stresses σ_{xx}, σ_{yy} with corresponding changes in (4.8):

$$
\begin{aligned}
\sigma_{xx} &= \frac{1}{2S_\triangle}\left[\frac{F_{012}+F_{016}}{a}a_xa_x + \frac{F_{023}+F_{021}}{b}b_xb_x + \frac{F_{034}+F_{032}}{c}c_xc_x\right] \\
&= \frac{1}{2\frac{\sqrt{3}}{4}x^2l_0^2}\left[2\frac{k_{al}l_0\frac{\sqrt{3}}{12}\frac{x^2-1}{x}}{xl_0}(\frac{\sqrt{3}}{2}xl_0)^2 + 2\frac{k_{al}l_0\frac{\sqrt{3}}{12}\frac{x^2-1}{x}}{xl_0}(-\frac{\sqrt{3}}{2}xl_0)^2\right] \\
&= \frac{2}{\sqrt{3}x^2l_0^2}\left[4\frac{k_{al}l_0\frac{\sqrt{3}}{12}\frac{x^2-1}{x}}{xl_0}(\frac{\sqrt{3}}{2}xl_0)^2\right] \\
&= \frac{2}{\sqrt{3}x^2l_0^2}\left[k_{al}\frac{\sqrt{3}}{3}\frac{x^2-1}{x^2}\frac{3}{4}x^2l_0^2\right] \\
&= k_{al}\frac{1}{2}\frac{x^2-1}{x^2} \\
\sigma_{yy} &= \frac{1}{2S_\triangle}\left[\frac{F_{012}+F_{016}}{a}a_ya_y + \frac{F_{023}+F_{021}}{b}b_yb_y + \frac{F_{034}+F_{032}}{c}c_yc_y\right] \\
&= \frac{1}{2\frac{\sqrt{3}}{4}x^2l_0^2}\left[2\frac{k_{al}l_0\frac{\sqrt{3}}{12}\frac{x^2-1}{x}}{xl_0}(\frac{1}{2}xl_0)^2 + 2\frac{k_{al}l_0\frac{\sqrt{3}}{12}\frac{x^2-1}{x}}{xl_0}(xl_0)^2\right. \\
&\quad \left. +2\frac{k_{al}l_0\frac{\sqrt{3}}{12}\frac{x^2-1}{x}}{xl_0}(\frac{1}{2}xl_0)^2\right] \\
&= \frac{2}{\sqrt{3}x^2l_0^2}2\frac{k_{al}l_0\frac{\sqrt{3}}{12}\frac{x^2-1}{x}}{xl_0}\left[(\frac{1}{2}xl_0)^2 + (xl_0)^2 + (\frac{1}{2}xl_0)^2\right] \\
&= \frac{1}{x^2l_0^2}k_{al}\frac{1}{3}\frac{x^2-1}{x^2}\left[\frac{3}{2}x^2l_0^2\right] \\
&= k_{al}\frac{1}{2}\frac{x^2-1}{x^2}. \tag{D.7}
\end{aligned}
$$

By analogous derivation, we continue with three-body interactions involving global area force. Exploiting the similarity with local area force we can directly write

$$
\sigma_{xx} = k_{ag}\frac{1}{2}(x^2-1), \quad \sigma_{yy} = k_{ag}\frac{1}{2}(x^2-1).
$$

After these tedious computations, we arrived at the expression for diagonal pressure:

$$
\begin{aligned}
P &= \frac{1}{2}(2k_s\sqrt{3}\frac{x-1}{x} + 2k_{al}\frac{1}{2}\frac{x^2-1}{x^2} + 2k_{ag}\frac{1}{2}(x^2-1)) \\
&= k_s\sqrt{3}\frac{x-1}{x} + \frac{k_{al}}{2}\frac{x^2-1}{x^2} + \frac{k_{ag}}{2}(x^2-1) \tag{D.8}
\end{aligned}
$$

using (D.3).

Further, we know that $A = cl_0^2 x^2$. Then we have

$$x = \frac{A^{1/2}}{c^{1/2}l_0}, \quad \frac{dx}{dA} = \frac{1}{2cxl_0^2}.$$

Using this relation in (D.2) we get

$$\frac{dP}{dA} = \frac{dP}{dx}\frac{dx}{dA} = \frac{dP}{dx}\frac{1}{2cxl_0^2} = \frac{dP}{dx}\frac{x}{2A_0}.$$

Putting all together we arrive at

$$\frac{dP}{dA}A_0 = \frac{dP}{dx}\frac{x}{2A_0}A_0 = \frac{dP}{dx}\frac{x}{2}.$$

We can now derive the relation for K:

$$K = A_0\left.\frac{dP}{d\log A}\right|_{A=A_0} = \left.\frac{dP}{dx}\frac{x}{2}\right|_{x=1}$$

$$= \left.\frac{x\,d(k_s\sqrt{3}\frac{x-1}{x} + \frac{k_{al}}{2}\frac{x^2-1}{x^2} + \frac{k_{ag}}{2}(x^2-1))}{2}\right|_{x=1}$$

$$= \left.\frac{x}{2}k_s\sqrt{3}\frac{1}{x^2}\right|_{x=1} + \left.\frac{x}{2}\frac{k_{al}}{2}\frac{2}{x^3}\right|_{x=1} + \left.\frac{x}{2}\frac{k_{ag}}{2}2x\right|_{x=1}$$

$$K = k_s\frac{\sqrt{3}}{2} + \frac{k_{al}}{2} + \frac{k_{ag}}{2}. \tag{D.9}$$

Before, we made a simplification for the formula for stretching forces. Instead of the non-linear formula (3.2) we considered its linear version $f_c = k_s(x-1)l_0$. If we do take into account the non-linearity $\kappa(x)$, the only difference would be that the term for differentiating will be more complicated and instead of differentiation

$$\left.\frac{d}{dx}\left(\frac{x-1}{x}\right)\right|_{x=1},$$

we need to differentiate

$$\left.\frac{d}{dx}\left(\kappa(x)\frac{x-1}{x}\right)\right|_{x=1} = \left.\frac{d}{dx}\left(\frac{x^{0.5} + x^{-2.5}}{x + x^{-3}}\frac{x-1}{x}\right)\right|_{x=1}.$$

Luckily, such a derivative evaluated at $x = 1$ turns out 1 in both cases.

D.3 Comment on differences in implementations of local area forces

In Section 4.2.4 we derive the relation between local area coefficient k_{al} and the area expansion modulus K. This links the parameter of the mesh to the physical quantity of the membrane. A similar relation has been derived for other models, too. Namely, for DPD model, the relation is identical up to a multiplicative constant 2. We comment on this in Section 4.2.4. Here we provide details explaining the difference.

To summarise, in the DPD model, the relation between local area coefficient k_d and area expansion modulus K is $K = k_d$, while in our IB-DC model, this relation reads as $K = k_{al}/2$. To see why this is so, let us compute DPD local area forces for an equilateral triangle. Denote $\mathbf{a}_{ij} = \mathbf{p}_i - \mathbf{p}_j$, where $\mathbf{p}_i$ are position vectors of the triangle vertices. The area of the deformed triangle is denoted by A and of the undeformed triangle by A_0. To evaluate the local area forces we use (A.4) in [56],

$$\mathbf{F}_{DPD} = \alpha \mathbf{N} \times \mathbf{a}_{32},$$

where $\mathbf{N} = \mathbf{a}_{21} \times \mathbf{a}_{31}$ and $\alpha = k_d(A - A_0)/(4A_0 A)$. Vectors $\mathbf{a}_{21}, \mathbf{a}_{32}, \mathbf{a}_{31}$ form an equilateral triangle so $|\mathbf{a}_{ij}| = xl_0$. Also, $A_k - A_0 = \Delta S_\triangle$ and $A_k = S_\triangle$. We can thus compute

$$|\mathbf{N}| = xl_0 \, xl_0 \sin(\pi/6) = x^2 l_0^2 \sqrt{3}/2.$$

Further computation reveals

$$|\mathbf{N} \times \mathbf{a}_{32}| = x^2 l_0^2 \sqrt{3}/2 \, xl_0 . \sin \pi/2 = x^3 l_0^3 \sqrt{3}/2.$$

Further from (D.4) we know that

$$\alpha = k_d \frac{A_k - A_0}{4A_0 A_k} = k_d \frac{\Delta S_\triangle}{4A_0 S_\triangle} = k_d \frac{\frac{\sqrt{3}}{4}(x^2 - 1)l_0^2}{4 \frac{\sqrt{3}}{4} l_0^2 \frac{\sqrt{3}}{4} x^2 l_0^2} = k_d \frac{(x^2 - 1)}{l_0^2 \sqrt{3} x^2}.$$

Altogether we get

$$|\mathbf{F}_{DPD}| = |\alpha||\mathbf{N} \times \mathbf{a}_{32}| = k_d \frac{(x^2 - 1)}{l_0^2 \sqrt{3} x^2} x^3 l_0^3 \sqrt{3}/2 = k_d \frac{(x^2 - 1)}{2} xl_0.$$

On the other hand, local area forces in our IB-DC model are given by (D.5) and further using (D.4) we end up with

$$|\mathbf{F}_{DC}| = k_{al} |\mathbf{T} - \mathbf{A}| \frac{\Delta S_\triangle}{t_a^2 + t_b^2 + t_c^2} = k_{al} \frac{1}{\sqrt{3}} xl_0 \frac{\frac{\sqrt{3}}{4}(x^2 - 1)l_0^2}{x^2 l_0^2} = k_{al} \frac{(x^2 - 1)}{4x} l_0.$$

The parameter for area expansion x vanishes when considering the limit case $x \to 0$. The remaining difference in denominators of both relations explains the multiplicative constant 2.

Appendix E

Complete example script

In Chapter 2, we have seen two versions of an introductory simulation script: a basic one, with just one cell and a more complex one, with two cells and a few obstacles. Here we present the same script one more time, in a version that looks closer to how a researcher might use it, even though we keep the scaled-down cells (radius of $r = 2\mu m$) and corresponding (non-physical) coefficients. Simulation parameters for regular red blood cells can be found in Appendix F.

- *Adding even more cells*

```
cell2 = oif.OifCell(cell_type=type, particle_type=?, origin=[?,?,?])
```

Their `particle_type` should be unique and they should be located somewhere, where they do not collide with existing cells or obstacles. The positions and rotations may be randomly generated.

- *Cell-wall interactions for the new cells*

```
system.non_bonded_inter[?,10].soft_sphere.set_params( \
a = 0.0001, n = 1.2, cutoff = 0.1, offset = 0.0)
```

Do not forget to specify the correct `particle_type` in the interaction. What will happen if you add more cells and use up all numbers from 0 to 9? Next is 10, of course, and thus the boundaries should get a different `particle_type`, anything higher than the largest one you used for cells.

- *Cell-cell interactions for the new cells*

```
system.non_bonded_inter[0,?].membrane_collision.set_params(\
a = 0.0001, n = 1.2, cutoff = 0.1, offset = 0.0)
system.non_bonded_inter[1,?].membrane_collision.set_params(\
a = 0.0001, n = 1.2, cutoff = 0.1, offset = 0.0)
```

Also interactions with existing cells are needed. Clearly, the number of these grows quadratically with number of cells and if you have more than a few cells, it makes sense to write these in a loop.

- *Automatic numbering of output folders*

```
cell2.output_vtk_pos_folded(file_name="output/sim3/cell2_" \
    + str(i) + ".vtk")
```

Here we have changed the output directory to *output/sim3*. It needs to be done in the whole script. Now is a good time to think ahead a little. After this simulation, there will likely come another one that should have output in *output/sim4*. Doing these changes manually in the script every time we want to run it again will not only be boring and error-prone, but extremely inefficient. It is a good thing we can automate that.

We replace "sim1" by "sim" + str(simNo). We already saw that str function changes numbers to strings and here the number will be a simulation number simNo. Instead of setting its value somewhere at the beginning of the script (which would still be a timesaver compared to our situation just a moment ago), we pass it as a parameter from the command line.

- *Passing arguments from command line*

```
sim_no = sys.argv[1]
os.makedirs("output/sim" + str(sim_no))
```

The first line sets the simulation number according to the command line argument and the second one creates a new directory inside the *output* folder with this number. The command line to run the simulation is ./pypresso script.py 4, where the 4 is the current simulation number.

Also, the simulations do not have to be identified by numbers. The folder can be called by what it actually contains (e.g. sim_with_one_cell and sim_with_two_cells), where we pass the string as a parameter. We do not have to pass just a single parameter from the command line. Some of other frequently used parameters are number of red blood cells, boolean variable for whether we want a graphical output, etc.

- *Separate method for creating boundaries*
  For clarity, It is useful to isolate the creation of boundaries into a separate method or alternatively, they could be read from a file.

- *Poisseuille flow in ESPResSo*
  In ESPResSo, we can move the fluid by creating a rhomboid boundary and setting the velocity on its boundary. This however sets a constant velocity over some surface. When we set this type of boundary, e.g. on the left inflow of the pipe, the fluid has a constant profile of the velocity and not the parabolic profile, as it is in Poisseuille flow. The parabolic profile develops by itself at a certain distance from the inflow.

An alternative option is to specify uniform force per unit of volume (lbf ext_force) and let the flow develop. The magnitude of this force may be tuned to achieve the desired maximal velocity in the center of the channel.

Here is the simulation script one more time, after all of these modifications:

```
import espressomd
import object_in_fluid as oif
from espressomd import lb
from espressomd import lbboundaries
from espressomd import shapes
from espressomd import interactions
import numpy as np
import os, sys, random

def create_obstacles():
    # bottom of the channel
    tmp_shape = shapes.Rhomboid(corner=[0.0, 0.0, 0.0], \
    a=[boxX, 0.0, 0.0], b=[0.0, boxY, 0.0], c=[0.0, 0.0, 1.0], direction=1)
    boundaries.append(tmp_shape)
    oif.output_vtk_rhomboid(rhom_shape=tmp_shape, \
    out_file=vtk_directory + "/wallBottom.vtk")

    # top of the channel
    tmp_shape = shapes.Rhomboid(corner=[0.0, 0.0, boxZ - 1], \
    a=[boxX, 0.0, 0.0], b=[0.0, boxY, 0.0], c=[0.0, 0.0, 1.0], direction=1)
    boundaries.append(tmp_shape)
    oif.output_vtk_rhomboid(rhom_shape=tmp_shape, \
    out_file=vtk_directory + "/wallTop.vtk")

    # front wall of the channel
    tmp_shape = shapes.Rhomboid(corner=[0.0, 0.0, 0.0], \
    a=[boxX, 0.0, 0.0], b=[0.0, 1.0, 0.0], c=[0.0, 0.0, boxZ], direction=1)
    boundaries.append(tmp_shape)
    oif.output_vtk_rhomboid(rhom_shape=tmp_shape, \
    out_file=vtk_directory + "/wallFront.vtk")

    # back wall of the channel
    tmp_shape = shapes.Rhomboid(corner=[0.0, boxY - 1.0, 0.0], \
    a=[boxX, 0.0, 0.0], b=[0.0, 1.0, 0.0], c=[0.0, 0.0, boxZ], direction=1)
    boundaries.append(tmp_shape)
    oif.output_vtk_rhomboid(rhom_shape=tmp_shape, \
    out_file=vtk_directory + "/wallBack.vtk")

    # obstacle - cylinder A
    centerA = [11.0, 2.0, boxZ/2]
    cyl_centers.append(centerA)
    tmp_shape = shapes.Cylinder(center=centerA, axis=[0.0, 0.0, 1.0], \
```

```
              length=boxZ, radius=cyl_radius, direction=1)
          boundaries.append(tmp_shape)
          oif.output_vtk_cylinder(cyl_shape=tmp_shape, n=20, \
          out_file=vtk_directory + "/cylinderA.vtk")

          # obstacle - cylinder B
          centerB = [16.0, 8.0, boxZ/2]
          cyl_centers.append(centerB)
          tmp_shape = shapes.Cylinder(center=centerB, axis=[0.0, 0.0, 1.0], \
          length=boxZ, radius=cyl_radius, direction=1)
          boundaries.append(tmp_shape)
          oif.output_vtk_cylinder(cyl_shape=tmp_shape, n=20, \
          out_file=vtk_directory + "/cylinderB.vtk")

          # obstacle - cylinder C
          centerC = [11.0, 12.0, boxZ/2]
          cyl_centers.append(centerC)
          tmp_shape = shapes.Cylinder(center=centerC, axis=[0.0, 0.0, 1.0], \
          length=boxZ, radius=cyl_radius, direction=1)
          boundaries.append(tmp_shape)
          oif.output_vtk_cylinder(cyl_shape=tmp_shape, n=20, \
          out_file=vtk_directory + "/cylinderC.vtk")

# find distance to the closest obstacle
def dist_to_closest_obstacle (x,y):
    min_dist = 100000000.0
    for center in cyl_centers:
        dist = oif.vec_distance([center[0], center[1], 0], [x, y, 0])
        if dist < min_dist:
            min_dist = dist
    if min_dist < cyl_radius + rbc_radius:
        min_dist = 0
    else:
        min_dist = min_dist - cyl_radius - rbc_radius
    return min_dist

if len(sys.argv)!= 3:
    print "2 arguments are expected:"
    print "number of cells: n_cells"
    print "id of the simulation: sim_no"
    print " "
else:
    n_cells = int(sys.argv[1])
    sim_no = sys.argv[2]

directory = "output/sim"+str(sim_no)
os.makedirs(directory)
vtk_directory = directory+"/vtk"
os.makedirs(vtk_directory)
```

```
boxX = 22.0
boxY = 14.0
boxZ = 14.0
system = espressomd.System(box_l=[boxX, boxY, boxZ])
system.cell_system.skin = 0.2
system.time_step = 0.1

cyl_radius = 2.0
cyl_centers = list()
boundaries = []
create_obstacles()
rbc_radius = 2.0

# random seeding of cells
cell_positions = list()
for k in range(0,n_cells):
    origin_ok = 0
    while origin_ok !=1:
        # generate random position in channel;
        ox = random.random() * (boxX - 2*rbc_radius) + rbc_radius
        oy = random.random() * (boxY - 2*rbc_radius - 2) + 1 + rbc_radius
        oz = random.random() * (boxZ - 2*rbc_radius - 2) + 1 + rbc_radius
        origin_ok = 1

        # check whether cells are outside of obstacles
        if dist_to_closest_obstacle(ox, oy) < 1:
            origin_ok = 0

        # check that it does not collide with other rbc
        if origin_ok == 1:
            for i in range(0,k):
                dist = oif.vec_distance([ox, oy, oz], cell_positions[i])
                if dist < 2*rbc_radius:
                    origin_ok = 0
                    break

        # if everything was ok, remember origin
        if origin_ok == 1:
            print ("seeding cell: "+str(k)+" with origin: "+str(ox)+", \
            "+str(oy)+", "+str(oz))
            cell_positions.append([ox,oy,oz])

# creating the template for RBCs
type = oif.OifCellType(nodes_file="input/rbc374nodes.dat", \
triangles_file="input/rbc374triangles.dat", check_orientation=False, \
system=system, ks=0.02, kb=0.016, kal=0.02, kag=0.9, kv=0.5, \
normal=True, resize=[rbc_radius, rbc_radius, rbc_radius])
```

```
# creating the RBCs
rbcs = list()
for id, pos in enumerate(cell_positions):
    cell_rbc = oif.OifCell(cell_type=type, particle_type=id, origin=pos,
    rotate=[random.random()*2*np.pi, random.random()*2*np.pi,
    random.random()*2*np.pi], particle_mass=0.5)
    rbcs.append(cell_rbc)
for id, rbc in enumerate(rbcs):
    rbc.output_vtk_pos(vtk_directory+"/rbc"+str(id)+".vtk")

# fluid
lbf = espressomd.lb.LBFluid(agrid=1, dens=1.0, visc=1.5, \
tau=system.time_step, fric=1.5, ext_force=[0.002, 0.0, 0.0])
system.actors.add(lbf)

# creating boundaries
for boundary in boundaries:
    system.lbboundaries.add(lbboundaries.LBBoundary(shape=boundary))
    system.constraints.add(shape=boundary, particle_type=100, penetrable=0)

# cell-wall interactions
for i in range(n_cells):
    system.non_bonded_inter[i, 100].soft_sphere.set_params(a=0.0001, \
    n=1.2, cutoff=0.1, offset=0.0)

# cell-cell interactions
system.non_bonded_inter[0, 1].membrane_collision.set_params(a=0.0001, \
n=1.2, cutoff=0.1, offset=0.0)
for i in range(n_cells):
    for j in range (n_cells):
        if (i<j):
            system.non_bonded_inter[i, j].membrane_collision.set_params(\
            a=0.0001, n=1.2, cutoff=0.1, offset=0.0)

# main integration loop
maxCycle = 100
for i in range(1, maxCycle):
    system.integrator.run(steps=500)
    for id, rbc in enumerate(rbcs):
        rbc.output_vtk_pos_folded(file_name=vtk_directory + "/cell" \
        + str(id) + "_" + str(i) + ".vtk")
    print "time: ", str(i*system.time_step)
print "Simulation completed."
```

Things to ponder

What happens, when you accidentally enter the same simulation number again, i.e. the directory already exists?

And maybe it is not even an accident. If the original script had a typo somewhere, it crashed with an error message, but the directory was already created. You would like to have it replaced with a new one with the same number with some actual output in it. How would you modify the script to be able to do that?

Appendix F

Simulation setup

To properly set up a simulation, we need to pay attention to the various parameters.

F.1   Units

Typically, for blood cell simulations, the micrometer scale is reasonable, since the diameter of a red blood cell is about $7.82\mu m = 7.82 \times 10^{-6} m$. The units used in models are called lattice units (typically denoted by L) and for the diameter of a red blood cell, this would mean $r_{RBC} = 7.82 Lm$. Note that while some simulation packages have a predefined unit system, ESPResSo does not and therefore the user is responsible for selecting a scaling, making sure the selected units are reasonable for the modeled system and that all physical quantities are scaled accordingly. One possible scaling can be defined as follows:

Basic scaling

- length: $1m = 10^6 Lm$

- time: $1s = 10^6 Ls$

- mass: $1kg = 10^{15} Lkg$

With these three, it is possible to derive the lattice units of all other physical quantities that are now uniquely determined. For example density has the IS unit kg/m^3. To convert it to lattice units, we do the following: $kg/m^3 = 10^{15} Lkg/10^{18} Lm^3 = 10^{-3} Lkg/Lm^3$. Therefore, if we wanted to use the density $20kg/m^3$, the simulation variable would be set as *density* $= 0.02$.

Other physical quantities in basic scaling

- density: $1kg/m^3 = 10^{-3}Lkg/Lm^3$
- kinematic viscosity: $1m^2/s = 10^6 Lm^2/Ls$
- force: $1N = 1kgm/s^2 = 10^9 LkgLm/Ls^2$
- pressure: $1kgm^{-1}s^{-2} = 10^{-3}LkgLm^{-1}Ls^{-2}$
- velocity: $1m/s = 1Lm/Ls$
- stretching coefficient: $1N/m = 1kg/s^2 = 10^3 Lkg/Ls^2$
- force density: $1Pa/m = 1kgm^{-2}s^{-2} = 10^{-9}LPa/Lm$

Note, that this is the scaling we are using throughout this book and in all scripts unless noted otherwise. Could we then take completely *arbitrary* scaling by fixing length, time and mass and figuring out lattice units for all other quantities? No. It is important to recognize that besides the physical constraints there might be numerical constraints as well. An example is the LBM which only reproduces the correct hydrodynamic interactions in a certain parameter range. More explanation of scaling can be found in [109].

An example of alternative scaling one might consider, is the following where the time *runs 10 times faster* compared to the basic scaling. This might be useful for the simulation of slow processes.

Alternative scaling

- length: $1m = 10^6 Lm$
- time: $1s = 10^5 Ls$
- mass: $1kg = 10^{15}Lkg$

Other physical quantities in alternative scaling

- density: $1kg/m^3 = 10^{-3}Lkg/Lm^3$
- kinematic viscosity: $1m^2/s = 10^7 Lm^2/Ls$
- force: $1N = 1kgm/s^2 = 10^{11}LkgLm/Ls^2$
- pressure: $1kgm^{-1}s^{-2} = 10^{-1}LkgLm^{-1}Ls^{-2}$
- velocity: $1m/s = 10Lm/Ls$
- stretching coefficient: $1N/m = 1kg/s^2 = 10^5 Lkg/Ls^2$

- force density: $1Pa/m = 1kgm^{-2}s^{-2} = 10^{-7}LPa/Lm$

Things to ponder
How does doubling of the space discretisation (i.e. $\Delta x = 2\mu m$ instead of $\Delta x = 1\mu m$) change scaling? What is the reduction in number of lattice nodes (and thus is computation time for the fluid) in this case?

F.2 Calculation of membrane coefficients

- *Stretching:* Using the formula (4.10) and the values of shear modulus reported from experiments [186], we can calculate the stretching coefficient $k_s = 5.5 \times 4/\sqrt{3}\mu N/m = 12.7\mu N/m$. Using the standard scaling, this translates into $k_s = 0.0127$ in our model.

- *Area compression/expansion:* For local area coefficient, we consider the issues discussed in Section 4.2.4 and set $k_{al} = 2k_s = 0.0254$ and k_{ag} to correspond to $K = 0.4N/m$, i.e. $k_{ag} = 800$ in standard scaling. Note that the value $k_{ag} = 800$ might be too large from a numerical perspective and therefore for practical purposes it makes sense to make k_{ag} just large enough that the total surface of the simulated cell does not change above a predefined threshold, e.g. 1% deviation. In the calibration simulations it was observed that the value $k_{ag} = 0.5$.

- *Viscosity:* Using the formula and measured values provided in Section 4.2.4, we calculate the viscosity coefficient $\gamma^C = 0.005 \times 4/\sqrt{3}\mu N \ s/m = 0.0115\mu Ns/m$, which translates into $k_{visc} = 11.5$ in standard scaling.

- *Bending:* Using the formula and measured values provided in Section 4.2.4, we calculate $k_b = \sqrt{3} \times 1.15 \times 10^{-19}Nm \sim 2 \times 10^{-19}Nm$, which is $k_b = 0.0002$ in our model in standard scaling.

- *Volume conservation:* The volume coefficient is chosen purely to maintain the volume of the cell and to have minimal deviation of the volume under 1%. In the calibration simulations, it was observed that the value $k_v = 0.9$ is sufficient.

Note, that these values were calculated under some assumptions, which do not hold exactly for our meshes and therefore a subsequent calibration is needed that can treat them as starting points. An example set of coefficients that fit the optical tweezers stretching experiment is $k_s = 0.006, k_b = 0.008, k_{al} = 0.001, k_{ag} = 0.5, k_v = 0.9$.

F.3 Determining friction coefficient and mesh densities

- *Red blood cell with 393 nodes (RBC_{393}):* Using the results from Table 3.4 and formula (3.20), for simulations of cells with radius $\sim 4\mu m$ in blood plasma, we can use the value $\xi = 1.82 \times \sqrt{135}/\sqrt{201} = 1.49$.

- *RBC_n:* If we want to use a red blood cell with different number of nodes, n, the friction coefficient is calculated using the formula $\xi_n = 1.49 \times 393/n$.

- *Another cell in simulation with RBC_{393}:* If there are other elastic objects in the simulation in addition to the red blood cell(s), e.g. a CTC as in Section 6.4, they will of course have the same friction coefficient as the RBC, since this is a global parameter for the whole simulation. In order for the CTC-fluid coupling to be correct then, we cannot choose arbitrary discretisation of the sphere that represents the CTC. The correct number of mesh nodes for CTC_m is then calculated using (3.20) as $m = 393 \times \sqrt{S_{CTC}}/\sqrt{S_{RBC}}$, where $S_{RBC} \sim 135$ (μm^2) is the surface area of the red blood cell (with radius $\sim 4\mu m$) and S_{CTC} is the surface area the CTC (other cell).

- *Another type of cell:* If we want to perform a simulation with another type of cell, we use (3.20) to determine the friction coefficient.

Note that these calculations are based on the sphere reference value $\xi = 1.82$ that was obtained at fluid density 1.025 and dynamic fluid viscosity 1.54. If one wants to use different viscosity, the friction coefficient should be adjusted, e.g. by linear interpolation using the values provided in Table 3.4. With increasing viscosity, the friction coefficient increases as well. It can also be shown that the friction coefficient increases with increasing density. These values are independent of the mass of immersed boundary points and it is recommended to set the mass to the membrane mass divided by the number of mesh points.

F.4 Setting up interactions

- *Cell-wall interactions:* To determine the coefficients of the soft-sphere cell-wall interaction, we can run a simulation with a cell in flow with an obstacle. We let the cell hit the obstacle and observe the deformation and the gap between the cell and the obstacle, as in Figure F.1. We fine-tune the interaction parameters so that the gap is minimal and deformation reasonable. The determined parameters are specific for the given flow velocity, so the calibration has to be repeated for different velocities. For larger velocities, the parameters increase, for lower velocities, they decrease. An example parameter set for an RBC-wall interaction is $a_{soft} = 0.0003$, $n_{soft} = 1.2$, $cut_{soft} = 0.1$ for $|\mathbf{v}_{max}| = 0.0007$. The maximum velocity was measured after the flow has developed in the chamber without the cell.

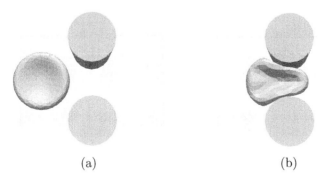

(a)   (b)

FIGURE F.1: Example setup for calibrating the cell-wall interaction. (a) Initial cell position. (b) Interaction coefficients must be set to such values that the cell touches the obstacles when passing through constriction.

- *Cell-cell interactions:* The approach is similar to the cell-wall interactions, but this time it is two elastic objects that interact instead of one solid and one elastic object. We let the two cells collide (e.g. in flow with an obstacle that stands in their way as in Figure F.2) and observe their deformation and the gap between them. We fine-tune the interaction parameters so that the gap is minimal. The determined parameters are again specific for the given flow velocity. An example parameter set for RBC-RBC interaction is $a_{membrane} = 0.03$, $n_{membrane} = 2.5$, $cut_{membrane} = 0.2$ for $|\mathbf{v}_{max}| = 0.0004$.

A few things to note:

- The maximum velocity was again measured after the flow has developed in the chamber without the cells.
- If one of the cells is stiffer (e.g. a CTC), the parameters have to reflect that.
- The cells are not aligned with the cylindrical obstacle exactly. If we did that, the symmetry of the setup would add another artificial property to an already very unphysical situation.

- *Order:* The order in which the individual model components are specified in a script has an impact on speed. Some of them cannot be specified

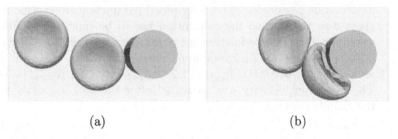

(a)   (b)

FIGURE F.2: Example setup for calibrating the cell-cell interaction. (a) Initial setup. (b) Interaction coefficients must be set to such values that the cells touch but the membranes do not intersect when in contact.

before others (e.g. cells before cell types), but some can (e.g. fluid boundaries before fluid), even though it is not recommended. The proper order is as follows:

- cell types
- cells
- cell-cell interactions
- fluid
- fluid boundaries
- cell-wall interactions

If cell types and cells are specified after the fluid, the simulation is slower. Interactions can only be defined once both the objects and boundaries exist. The cell-cell interactions can also be specified at a later point.

F.5 Fluid parameters

- *Density of blood plasma:* $\rho = 1025 kgm^{-3}$, which is 1.025 in our scaling.

- *Dynamic viscosity of human blood plasma:* at $37°C$ is $1.34 \times 10^{-3} Pas$, which is 1.34 in our scaling. Due to the immersed blood cells, the viscosity of whole blood when considered as a homogeneous fluid is $3 - 4 \times 10^{-3} Pas$.

- *Kinematic viscosity of blood plasma:* at $37°C$ is $1.34/1.025 \times 10^{-6} m^2/s$, which is 1.31 in our scaling. Note that the viscosity increases with decreasing temperature. Kinematic viscosity is the one we use in ESPResSo.

- *Typical velocities in microfluidic devices:* Note that in simulation we do not prescribe velocities, but rather fluid forces which are adjusted to give the correct maximum velocities as measured in the central parts of the channel. The experimentally measured maximum velocities in microfluidic devices vary from around 0.007-$0.008m/s$ in [19] to 0.017-$0.018m/s$ in [50].

Bibliography

[1] L. Abdelmohsen, F. Peng, Y. Tu, and D. Wilson. Micro- and nano-motors for biomedical applications. *Journal of Materials Chemistry B*, 2:2395–2408, 2014. (Cited on page 194.)

[2] M. Abkarian, M. Faivre, R. Horton, K. Smistrup, K. A. Best-Popescu, and H. A. Stone. Cellular-scale hydrodynamics. *Biomedical Materials*, 3:67–73, 2008. (Cited on page 118.)

[3] P. Ahlrichs and B. Dunweg. Lattice-Boltzmann simulation of polymer-solvent systems. *International Journal of Modern Physics C*, 8:1429–1438, 1998. (Cited on pages 48, 49, and 50.)

[4] B. Alberts, J. Watson, D. Bray, and J. Lewis. *Molecular Biology of the Cell*. Taylor & Francis (Garland Publishing), 2008. (Cited on page 25.)

[5] R. Alon, S. Chen, K. D. Puri, E. B. Finger, and T. A. Springer. The kinetics of L-selectin tethers and the mechanics of selectin-mediated rolling. *The Journal of Cell Biology*, 138(5):1169–1180, 1997. (Cited on pages 180 and 182.)

[6] A. Andren, A. R. Brown, P. J. Mason, J. Graf, U. Schumann, C.-H. Moeng, and F. T. M. Nieuwstadt. Large-eddy simulation of a neutrally stratified boundary layer: A comparison of four computer codes. *Quarterly Journal of the Royal Meteorological Society*, 120(520):1457–1484, 1994. (Cited on page 79.)

[7] A. Arnold, O. Lenz, S. Kesselheim, R. Weeber, F. Fahrenberger, D. Roehm, P. Košovan, and C. Holm. ESPResSo 3.1 - molecular dynamics software for coarse–grained models. In M. Griebel and M.A. Schweitzer, editors, *Meshfree Methods for Partial Differential Equations VI, Lecture Notes in Computational Science and Engineering*, volume 89, pages 1–23, 2013. (Cited on pages 8 and 187.)

[8] Scootdive at English Wikipedia. Published under the Creative Commons Attribution-Share Alike 3.0 Unported licence, https://creativecommons.org/licenses/by-sa/3.0/deed.en. Original figure was transformed into the greyscale, cut and an overlay graphics was added. Original figure available at

https://commons.wikimedia.org/wiki/File:Red_blood_cells_(2).jpg. (Cited on page 27.)

[9] K. Bachratá, H. Bachratý, and M. Slavík. Statistics for comparison of simulations and experiments of flow of blood cells. *EPJ Web of Conferences*, 143:02002, 2017. (Cited on page 123.)

[10] H. Bachratý, K. Kovalčíková, K. Bachratá, and M. Slavík. Methods of exploring the red blood cells rotation during the simulations in devices with periodic topology. In *2017 International Conference on Information and Digital Technologies (IDT)*, pages 36–46, 2017. (Cited on page 123.)

[11] J. S. Bagnall, S. Byun, S. Begum, D. T. Miyamoto, V. C. Hecht, S. Maheswaran, S. L. Stott, M. Toner, R. O. Hynes, and S. R. Manalis. Deformability of tumor cells versus blood cells. *Scientific Reports*, 5:ID 18542, 2015. (Cited on page 119.)

[12] A. V. Belyaev. Published under the Attribution 4.0 International (CC BY 4.0) licence, https://creativecommons.org/licenses/by/4.0/. Original figure was transformed into the greyscale. Original figure available at https://doi.org/10.1371/journal.pone.0183093. (Cited on page 175.)

[13] A. V. Belyaev. Hydrodynamic repulsion of spheroidal microparticles from micro-rough surfaces. *PLoS ONE*, 12(8):e0183093, 2017. (Cited on pages 174 and 175.)

[14] A. L. Blumers, Y. H. Tang, Z. Li, X. J. Li, and G. E. Karniadakis. GPU-accelerated red blood cells simulations with transport dissipative particle dynamics. *Computer Physics Communications*, 217:171–179, 2017. (Cited on page 76.)

[15] D. Boal. *Mechanics of the Cell*. Cambridge University Press, 2001. (Cited on pages 90, 98, and 183.)

[16] J. M. Bower. Looking for Newton: Realistic modeling in modern biology. *Brains, Minds and Media*, 1, 2005. (Cited on page xi.)

[17] D. E. Brooks, J. W. Goodwin, and G. V. Seaman. Interactions among erythrocytes under shear. *Journal of Applied Physiology*, 28(2):172–177, 1970. (Cited on page 63.)

[18] E. Buckingham. On physically similar systems; Illustrations of the use of dimensional equations. *Physical Review*, 4:345–376, 1914. (Cited on page 74.)

[19] D. M. Bukowska, L. Derzsi, S. Tamborski, M. Szkulmowski, P. Garstecki, and M. Wojtkowski. Assessment of the flow velocity of blood cells in a

microfluidic device using joint spectral and time domain optical coherence tomography. *Optics Express*, 21(20):24025–24038, 2013. (Cited on pages 159 and 241.)

[20] M. Bušík. H. Lee Moffitt Cancer Center and Research Institute, Tampa, Florida, USA, unpublished work. (Cited on page 188.)

[21] M. Bušík and I. Cimrák. The calibration of fluid-object interaction in immersed boundary method. *EPJ Web of Conferences*, 143:ID 02013, 2017. (Cited on pages 52, 54, 56, and 58.)

[22] M. Bušík, I. Jančigová, R. Tóthová, and I. Cimrák. Simulation study of rare cell trajectories and capture rate in periodic obstacle arrays. *Journal of Computational Science*, 17(2):370–376, 2016. (Cited on pages 156 and 159.)

[23] M. Bušík, M. Slavík, and I. Cimrák. Fluid-structure interaction by dissipative coupling in cell flow modeling. under review. (Cited on pages 57 and 59.)

[24] S. Byun, S. Son, D. Amodei, N. Cermak, J. Shaw, J. H. Kang, V. C. Hecht, M. M. Winslow, T. Jacks, P Mallick, and S. R. Manalis. Characterizing deformability and surface friction of cancer cells. *Proceedings of the National Academy of Sciences*, 110(19):7580–7585, 2013. (Cited on page 186.)

[25] H. Casquero, C. Bona-Casas, and H. Gomez. NURBS-based numerical proxies for red blood cells and circulating tumor cells in microscale blood flow. *Computer Methods in Applied Mechanics and Engineering*, 316:646–667, 2017. (Cited on pages 183 and 186.)

[26] S. Chen and G. D. Doolen. Lattice-Boltzmann method for fluid flows. *Annual Review of Fluid Mechanics*, 30:329–364, 1998. (Cited on page 47.)

[27] S. Chen and T. A. Springer. Selectin receptor–ligand bonds: Formation limited by shear rate and dissociation governed by the bell model. *Proceedings of the National Academy of Sciences*, 98(3):950–955, 2001. (Cited on page 180.)

[28] S. Chien and K. Jan. Ultrastructural basis of the mechanism of rouleaux formation. *Microvascular Research*, 5:155–166, 1973. (Cited on page 63.)

[29] C. D. Chin, V. Linder, and S. K. Sia. Commercialization of microfluidic point-of-care diagnostic devices. *Lab on a Chip*, 12:2118–2134, 2012. (Cited on page 150.)

[30] A. T. Chwang and T. Y-T. Wu. Hydromechanics of low-Reynolds-number flow. Part 2. Singularity method for Stokes flows. *Journal of Fluid Mechanics*, 67(4):787–815, 1975. (Cited on page 57.)

[31] I. Cimrák, M. Gusenbauer, and I. Jančigová. An ESPResSo implementation of elastic objects immersed in a fluid. *Computer Physics Communications*, 185(3):900–907, 2014. (Cited on pages 4, 8, and 76.)

[32] I. Cimrák, M. Gusenbauer, and T. Schrefl. Modelling and simulation of processes in microfluidic devices for biomedical applications. *Computers and Mathematics with Applications*, 64(3):278–288, 2012. (Cited on page 4.)

[33] J. R. Clausen, D. A. Reasor, and C. K. Aidun. Parallel performance of a lattice-Boltzmann/finite element cellular blood flow solver on the IBM Blue Gene/P architecture. *Computer Physics Communications*, 181:1013–1020, 2010. (Cited on pages 132 and 147.)

[34] A. Coclite, M. D. de Tullio, G. Pascazio, and P. Decuzzi. A combined lattice Boltzmann and Immersed Boundary approach for predicting the vascular transport of differently shaped particles. *Computers and Fluids*, 136:260–271, 2016. (Cited on page 188.)

[35] G. R. Cokelet and H. J. Meiselman. Rheological comparison of hemoglobin solutions and erythrocyte suspensions. *Science*, 162:275–277, 1968. (Cited on page 72.)

[36] E. Coumans. Bullet physics library. http://bulletphysics.org/, 2017. (Cited on page 136.)

[37] National Research Council. *Assessing the Reliability of Complex Models: Mathematical and Statistical Foundations of Verification, Validation, and Uncertainty Quantification*. The National Academies Press, Washington, DC, 2012. (Cited on page 78.)

[38] G. Cuce and T. M. Aktan. Platelets, 2012. Blood Cell, Terry E. Moschandreou, IntechOpen, Available from: https://www.intechopen.com/books/blood-cell-an-overview-of-studies-in-hematology/platelets,. (Cited on page 119.)

[39] Y. Dai, Y. Fu, H. Zeng, L. Xing, Y. Zhang, Y. Zhan, and X. Xue. A self-powered brain-linked vision electronic-skin based on triboelectric-photodetecting pixel-addressable matrix for visual-image recognition and behavior intervention. *Advanced Functional Materials*, 28(20), 2018. (Cited on page 193.)

[40] M. Dao, J. Li, and S. Suresh. Molecularly based analysis of deformation of spectrin network and human erythrocyte. *Materials Science and Engineering C*, 26:1232–1244, 2006. (Cited on pages 59, 70, 89, 95, 98, 101, 107, 108, and 219.)

[41] J. de Graaf, T. Peter, L. P. Fischer, and C. Holm. The raspberry model for hydrodynamic interactions revisited. ii. The effect of confinement.

Journal of Chemical Physics, 143:084108, 2015. (Cited on pages 50 and 187.)

[42] E. de Miguel and G. Jackson. The nature of the calculation of the pressure in molecular simulations of continuous models from volume perturbations. *Journal of Chemical Physics*, 125(16):164109, 2006. (Cited on page 92.)

[43] P. Decuzzi and M. Ferrari. The adhesive strength of non-spherical particles mediated by specific interactions. *Biomaterials*, 27(30):5307–5314, 2006. (Cited on pages 155, 156, and 157.)

[44] S. Deutsch, J. M. Tarbell, K. B. Manning, G. Rosenberg, and A. A. Fontaine. Experimental fluid mechanics of pulsatile artificial blood pumps. *Annual Review of Fluid Mechanics*, 38:65–86, 2006. (Cited on page 169.)

[45] P. Dimitrakopoulos. Analysis of the variation in the determination of the shear modulus of the erythrocyte membrane: Effects of the constitutive law and membrane modeling. *Physical Review E*, 85(041917), 2012. (Cited on page 120.)

[46] C. Dong and X. X. Lei. Biomechanics of cell rolling: Shear flow, cell-surface adhesion, and cell deformability. *Journal of Biomechanics*, 33(1):35–43, 2000. (Cited on pages 182 and 183.)

[47] B. Dunweg and A. J. C. Ladd. Lattice-Boltzmann simulations of soft matter systems. *Advances in Polymer Science*, 221:89–166, 2009. (Cited on pages 49 and 51.)

[48] M. M. Dupin, I. Halliday, C. M. Care, and L. Alboul. Modeling the flow of dense suspensions of deformable particles in three dimensions. *Physical Review E, Statistical, nonlinear, and soft matter physics*, 75, 2007. (Cited on pages 33 and 37.)

[49] B. Dura, S. K. Dougan, M. Barisa, M. M. Hoehl, H. L. Lo, C. T. Ploegh, and J. Voldman. Profiling lymphocyte interactions at the single-cell level by microfluidic cell pairing. *Nature Communications*, 6(5940):4589–4594, 2015. (Cited on page 63.)

[50] J. B. Edel, E. K. Hill, and A. J. de Mello. Velocity measurement of particulate flow in microfluidic channels using single point confocal fluorescence detection. *Analyst*, 126(11):1953–1957, 2001. (Cited on pages 159 and 241.)

[51] E. Evans and Y.-C. Fung. Improved measurements of the erythrocyte geometry. *Microvascular Research*, 4(4):335–347, 1972. (Cited on page 26.)

[52] E. A. Evans. Bending resistance and chemically induced moments in membrane bilayers. *Biophysics Journal*, 14(12):923–931, 1974. (Cited on page 90.)

[53] E. A. Evans. Bending elastic modulus of red blood cell membrane derived from buckling instability in micropipet aspiration tests. *Biophysical Journal*, 43(1):27–30, 1983. (Cited on page 103.)

[54] E. A. Evans and R. M. Hochmuth. Membrane viscoelasticity. *Biophysical Journal*, 16(1):1–11, 1976. (Cited on page 103.)

[55] E. A. Evans, R. Waugh, and L. Melnik. Elastic area compressibility modulus of red cell membrane. *Biophysical Journal*, 16(6):585–595, 1976. (Cited on page 105.)

[56] D. Fedosov. *Multiscale modeling of blood flow and soft matter*. PhD thesis, Brown University, 2010. (Cited on pages 37, 69, 70, 89, 95, 101, 102, 104, 120, 207, 209, 210, 214, 217, and 226.)

[57] D. A. Fedosov, B. Caswell, and G. E. Karniadakis. A multiscale red blood cell model with accurate mechanics, rheology and dynamics. *Biophysical Journal*, 98(10):2215–2225, 2010. (Cited on page 74.)

[58] D. A. Fedosov, B. Caswell, and G. E. Karniadakis. Wall shear stress-based model for adhesive dynamics of red blood cells in malaria. *Biophysical Journal*, 100:2084–2093, 2011. (Cited on page 157.)

[59] D. A. Fedosov, B. Caswell, A. S. Popel, and G. E. Karniadakis. Blood flow and cell-free layer in microvessels. *Microcirculation*, 17:615–628, 2010. (Cited on page 84.)

[60] D. A. Fedosov, M. Peltomaki, and G. Gompper. Deformation and dynamics of red blood cells in flow through cylindrical microchannels. *Soft Matter*, 10:4258, 2014. (Cited on page 115.)

[61] S. E. Feller. Molecular dynamics simulations of lipid bilayers. *Current Opinion in Colloid and Interface Science*, 5:217–223, 2000. (Cited on page 69.)

[62] J. Feng, D. D. Joseph, and H. H. Hu. Direct simulation of initial value problems for the motion of solid bodies in a newtonian fluid. Part 2. Couette and Poiseuille flows. *Journal of Fluid Mechanics*, 277:271–301, 1994. (Cited on page 188.)

[63] Z. G. Feng and E. E. Michaelides. The immersed boundary-lattice Boltzmann method for solving fluid-particles interaction problems. *Journal of Computational Physics*, 195:602–628, 2004. (Cited on page 71.)

[64] L. P. Fischer, T. Peter, C. Holm, and J. de Graaf. The raspberry model for hydrodynamic interactions revisited. I. Periodic arrays of spheres and dumbbells. *Journal of Chemical Physics*, 143:084107, 2015. (Cited on pages 50 and 187.)

[65] T. M. Fischer. Tank-tread frequency of the red cell membrane: Dependence on the viscosity of the suspending medium. *Biophysics Journal*, 93:2007, 2553–2561. (Cited on pages 110, 112, and 113.)

[66] Blender Foundation. Blender. https://www.blender.org/about/, 2017. (Cited on page 136.)

[67] R. Fåhraeus and T. Lindqvist. The viscosity of blood in narrow capillary tubes. *American Journal of Physiology*, 96:562–568, 1931. (Cited on page 84.)

[68] C. S. Frenk, S. D. M. White, P. Bode, J. R. Bond, G. L. Bryan, R. Cen, H. M. P. Couchman, A. E. Evrard, N. Gnedin, A. Jenkins, A. M. Khokhlov, A. Klypin, J. F. Navarro, M. L. Norman, J. P. Ostriker, J. M. Owen, F.R. Pearce, U.-L. Pen, M. Steinmetz, P. A. Thomas, J. V. Villumsen, J. W. Wadsley, M. S. Warren, G. Xu, and G. Yepes. The Santa Barbara Cluster Comparison Project: A comparison of cosmological hydrodynamics solutions. *Astrophysical Journal*, 525(2):554, 1999. (Cited on page 79.)

[69] D. Frenkel and B. Smit. *Understanding Molecular Simulation*. Elsevier Inc., 2002. (Cited on page 145.)

[70] J. B. Freund. Numerical simulation of flowing blood cells. *Annual Review of Fluid Mechanics*, 46:67–95, 2014. (Cited on page 71.)

[71] E. Gabriel, G. E. Fagg, G. Bosilca, T. Angskun, J. J. Dongarra, J. M. Squyres, V. Sahay, P. Kambadur, B. Barrett, A. Lumsdaine, R. H. Castain, D. J. Daniel, R. L. Graham, and T. S. Woodall. Open MPI: Goals, concept, and design of a next generation MPI implementation. In *Proceedings, 11th European PVM/MPI Users' Group Meeting*, pages 97–104, 2004. (Cited on page 148.)

[72] T. C. Gasser and A. Grytsan. Biomechanical modeling the adaptation of soft biological tissue. *Current Opinion in Biomedical Engineering*, 1:71–77, 2017. (Cited on page 193.)

[73] S. Gekle. Strongly accelerated margination of active particles in blood flow. *Biophysical Journal*, 110:514–520, 2016. (Cited on page 76.)

[74] C. Geuzaine and J. F. Remacle. Gmsh: a three-dimensional finite element mesh generator with built-in pre- and post-processing facilities. *International Journal for Numerical Methods in Engineering*, 79(11):1309–1331, 2009. (Cited on pages 26, 57, and 141.)

[75] J. P. Gleghorn, E. D. Pratt, D. Denning, H. Liu, N. H. Bander, S. T. Tagawa, D. M. Nanus, P. A. Giannakakou, and B. J. Kirby. Capture of circulating tumor cells from whole blood of prostate cancer patients using geometrically enhanced differential immunocapture (GEDI) and a prostate-specific antibody. *Lab on the Chip*, 10:27–29, 2010. (Cited on page 163.)

[76] J. P. Gleghorn, J. P. Smith, and B. J. Kirby. Transport and collision dynamics in periodic asymmetric obstacle arrays: Rational design of microfluidic rare-cell immunocapture devices. *Physical Review E*, 88:032136, 2013. (Cited on pages 163, 164, and 165.)

[77] D. E. Golan and W. Veatch. Lateral mobility of band 3 in the human erythrocyte membrane studied by fluorescence photobleaching recovery: Evidence for control by cytoskeletal interactions. *Proceedings of the National Academy of Sciences*, 77(5):2537–2541, 1980. (Cited on page 103.)

[78] G. Gompper, T. Ihle, D. M. Kroll, and R. G. Winkler. Multi-particle collision dynamics: A particle-based mesoscale simulation approach to the hydrodynamics of complex fluids. *Advanced Computer Simulation Approaches for Soft Matter Sciences*, III:1–87, 2009. (Cited on page 70.)

[79] G. Gompper and D. M. Kroll. Random surface discretizations and the renormalization of the bending rigidity. *Journal de Physique*, 6(10):1305–1320, 1996. (Cited on page 103.)

[80] G. Gompper and M. Schick. *Soft Matter: Lipid Bilayers and Red Blood Cells*. Wiley, 2008. (Cited on pages 28 and 68.)

[81] D. R. Gossett, H. T. K. Tse, S. A. Lee, Y. Ying, A. G. Lindgren, O. O. Yang, J. Rao, A. T. Clark, and D. D. Carlo. Hydrodynamic stretching of single cells for large population mechanical phenotyping. *Proceedings of the National Academy of Sciences*, 109(20):7630–7635, 2012. (Cited on page 119.)

[82] A. Guckenberger and S. Gekle. Theory and algorithms to compute Helfrich bending forces: A review. *Journal of Physics: Condensed Matter*, 29(20):203001, 2017. (Cited on pages 44 and 90.)

[83] Q. Guo, S. Park, and H. Ma. Microfluidic micropipette aspiration for measuring the deformability of single cells. *Lab Chip*, 12:2687–2695, 2012. (Cited on pages 105 and 118.)

[84] M. Gusenbauer, R. Tóthová, G. Mazza, M. Brandl, T. Schrefl, I. Jančigová, and I. Cimrák. Published under the Attribution-NonCommercial 4.0 International (CC BY-NC 4.0) licence, https://creativecommons.org/licenses/by-nc/4.0/. Original figure was transformed into the greyscale. Original figure available at https://doi.org/10.1111/aor.13111. (Cited on page 170.)

[85] M. Gusenbauer, R. Tóthová, G. Mazza, M. Brandl, T. Schrefl, I. Jančigová, and I. Cimrák. Cell damage index as computational indicator for blood cell activation and damage. *Artificial Organs*, 2018. DOI:10.1111/aor.13111. (Cited on pages 169, 170, and 171.)

[86] M. A. Haidekker, A. G. Tsai, T. Brady, H. Y. Stevens, J. A. Frangos, E. Theodorakis, and M. Intaglietta. A novel approach to blood plasma viscosity measurement using fluorescent molecular rotors. *American Journal of Physiology-Heart and Circulatory Physiology*, 282:H1609–H1614, 2002. (Cited on page 59.)

[87] D. A. Hammer and S. M. Apte. Simulation of cell rolling and adhesion on surfaces in shear flow: General results and analysis of selectin-mediated neutrophil adhesion. *Biophysical Journal*, 63:35–57, 1992. (Cited on page 157.)

[88] L. Hatton and A. Roberts. How accurate is scientific software? *IEEE Transactions on Software Engineering*, 20(10):785–797, 1994. (Cited on page 79.)

[89] W. Helfrich. Elastic properties of lipid bilayers: Theory and possible experiments. *Zeitschrift f'ur Naturforschung C*, 28:693–703, 1973. (Cited on pages 73 and 90.)

[90] A. Henderson. ParaView guide, A Parallel Visualization Application. Technical report, Kitware Inc., 2007. (Cited on pages 12 and 18.)

[91] S. Henon, G. Lenormand, A. Richert, and F. Gallet. A new determination of the shear modulus of the human erythrocyte membrane using optical tweezers. *Biophysical Journal*, 76:1145–1151, 1999. (Cited on page 98.)

[92] R. M. Hochmuth and R. E. Waugh. Erythrocyte membrane elasticity and viscosity. *Annual Review of Physiology*, 49:209–219, 1987. (Cited on page 98.)

[93] R. M. Hochmuth, P. R. Worthy, and E. A. Evans. Red cell extensional recovery and the determination of membrane viscosity. *Biophysical Journal*, 26:101–114, 1979. (Cited on pages 91 and 103.)

[94] J. F. Hoffman. Questions for red blood cell physiologists to ponder in this millenium. *Blood Cells, Molecules, and Diseases*, 27(1):57–61, 2001. (Cited on page 191.)

[95] C. Holm, A. Arnold, O. Lenz, and S. Kesselheim. ESPResSo documentation, April 2018. http://espressomd.org/wordpress/documentation. (Cited on page 8.)

[96] B. Hong and Y. Zu. Detecting circulating tumor cells: Current challenges and new trends. *Theranostics*, 3(6):377–394, 2013. (Cited on page 163.)

[97] S. M. Hosseini and J. J. Feng. How malaria parasites reduce the deformability of infected red blood cells. *Biophysical Journal*, 103:1–10, 2012. (Cited on page 70.)

[98] H. W. Hou, Q. S. Li, G. Y. H. Lee, A. P. Kumar, C. N. Ong, and C. T. Lim. Deformability study of breast cancer cells using microfluidics. *Biomed Microdevices*, 11:557–564, 2009. (Cited on page 119.)

[99] C. Huang, S. M. Santana, H. Liu, N. H. Bander, B. G. Hawkins, and B. J. Kirby. Characterization of a hybrid dielectrophoresis and immunocapture microfluidic system for cancer cell capture. *Electrophoresis*, 34(20-21):2970–2979, 2013. (Cited on page 163.)

[100] Cell in-fluid research group. Group's webpage, September 2018. http://cell-in-fluid.fri.uniza.sk. (Cited on pages 8 and 19.)

[101] I. Jančigová. *Modeling elastic objects in fluid flow with biomedical applications*. PhD thesis, University of Žilina, 2015. (Cited on page 133.)

[102] I. Jančigová and I. Cimrák. Non-uniform force allocation for area preservation in spring network models. *International Journal for Numerical Methods in Biomedical Engineering*, 32(10):e02757–n/a, 2016. (Cited on pages 37 and 209.)

[103] M. Ju, S. S. Ye, B. Namgung, S. Cho, H. T. Low, H. L. Leo, and S. Kim. A review of numerical methods for red blood cell flow simulation. *Computer Methods in Biomechanics and Biomedical Engineering*, 18:130–140, 2015. (Cited on page 63.)

[104] G. Késmárky, P. Kenyeres, M. Rábai, and K. Tóth. Plasma viscosity: A forgotten variable. *Clinical Hemorheology and Microcirculation*, 39:243–246, 2008. (Cited on page 59.)

[105] Y. Kim and C. Peskin. Penalty immersed boundary method for an elastic boundary with mass. *Physics of Fluids*, 19:053103, 2007. (Cited on page 51.)

[106] C. B. Korn and U. S. Schwarz. Dynamic states of cells adhering in shear flow: From slipping to rolling. *Physical Review E*, 77:041904, 2008. (Cited on pages 157, 180, and 181.)

[107] T. Krueger. *Computer Simulation Study of Collective Phenomena in Dense Suspensions of Red Blood Cells under Shear*. PhD thesis, Max-Planck Institut, 2012. (Cited on pages 51, 52, 61, 70, 71, 103, 104, 115, 130, 132, 205, 210, 213, and 217.)

[108] T. Krueger, D. Holmes, and P. V. Coveney. Deformability-based red blood cell separation in deterministic lateral displacement devices - a simulation study. *Biomicrofluidics*, 8(5):054114, 2014. (Cited on page 153.)

[109] T. Krueger, H. Kusumaatmaja, A. Kuzmin, O. Shardt, G. Silva, and E. M. Viggen. *The Lattice Boltzmann Method*. Springer, 2016. (Cited on pages 29, 48, 75, and 236.)

[110] T. Krueger, F. Varnik, and D. Raabe. Efficient and accurate simulations of deformable particles immersed in a fluid using a combined immersed boundary lattice Boltzmann finite element method. *Computers and Mathematics with Applications*, 61:3485–3505, 2011. (Cited on page 76.)

[111] Electric Ant Lab. Scientific modelling and simulations, 2018. [Online; accessed 6-April-2018]. (Cited on page 76.)

[112] A. J. C. Ladd, R. Kekre, and J. E. Butler. Comparison of the static and dynamic properties of a semiflexible polymer using lattice Boltzmann and Brownian dynamics simulations. *Physical Review E*, 80:036704, 2009. (Cited on page 50.)

[113] L. Lanotte, J. Mauer, S. Mendez, D. A. Fedosov, J.-M. Fromental, V. Claveria, F. Nicoud, G. Gompper, and M. Abkarian. Red cells' dynamic morphologies govern blood shear thinning under microcirculatory flow conditions. *Proceedings of the National Academy of Sciences*, 113(47):13289–13294, 2016. (Cited on page 76.)

[114] G. Lenormand, S. Henon, A. Richert, J. Simeon, and F. Gallet. Direct measurement of the area expansion and shear moduli of the human red blood cell membrane skeleton. *Biophysical Journal*, 81:43–56, 2001. (Cited on pages 96 and 101.)

[115] L. B. Leverett, J. D. Hellums, C. P. Alfrey, and E. C. Lynch. Red blood cell damage by shear stress. *Biophysical Journal*, 12(3):257–273, 1972. (Cited on page 170.)

[116] H. Li and G. Lykotrafitis. Erythrocyte membrane model with explicit description of the lipid bilayer and the spectrin network. *Biophysical Journal*, 107(3):642–653, 2014. (Cited on pages 27 and 68.)

[117] H. Li, X. Ruan, W. Qian, and X. Fu. Numerical estimation of hemolysis from the point of view of signal and system. *Artificial Organs*, 38(12):1065–1075, 2014. (Cited on page 169.)

[118] J. Li, M. Dao, C. T. Lim, and S. Suresh. Spectrin-level modeling of the cytoskeleton and optical tweezers stretching of the erythrocyte. *Biophysical Journal*, 88:3707–3719, 2005. (Cited on page 68.)

[119] S-J. Liao. An analytic approximation of the drag coefficient for the viscous flow past a sphere. *International Journal of Non-Linear Mechanics*, 37(1):1 – 18, 2002. (Cited on page 51.)

[120] M. C. Lin. *Efficient Collision Detection for Animation and Robotics.* PhD thesis, University of California, Berkeley, 1993. (Cited on page 63.)

[121] B. Lincoln, H. M. Erickson, S. Schinkinger, F. Wottawah, D. Mitchell, S. Ulvick, C. Bilby, and J. Guck. Deformability-based flow cytometry. *Cytometry Part A*, 59A(2):203–209, 2004. (Cited on page 108.)

[122] O. Linderkamp and H. J. Meiselman. Geometric, osmotic, and membrane mechanical properties of density-separated human red cells. *Blood*, 59(6):1121–1127, 1982. (Cited on pages 91 and 103.)

[123] Y. Liu and W. K. Liu. Rheology of red blood cell aggregation by computer simulation. *Journal of Computational Physics*, 220:139–154, 2006. (Cited on pages 47, 68, and 188.)

[124] V. Lobaskin and B. Dunweg. A new model for simulating colloidal dynamics. *New Journal of Physics*, 6:54, 2004. (Cited on page 50.)

[125] R. M. MacMeccan. *Mechanistic effects of erythrocytes on platelet deposition in coronary thrombosis.* PhD thesis, Georgia Institute of Technology, 2007. (Cited on page 132.)

[126] G. Marcelli, K. H. Parker, and C. P. Winlovey. Thermal fluctuations of red blood cell membrane via a constant-area particle-dynamics model. *Biophysical Journal*, 89:2473–2480, 2005. (Cited on page 69.)

[127] G. Mazza. Department for Integrated Sensor Systems, Danube University Krems, in-house experiments, 2017. (Cited on page 122.)

[128] J. McGrath, M. Jimenez, and H. Bridle. Deterministic lateral displacement for particle separation: A review. *Lab on a Chip*, 14:4139–4158, 2014. (Cited on page 153.)

[129] H. J. Meiselman, E. A. Evans, and R. M. Hochmuth. Membrane mechanical properties of ATP-depleted human erythrocytes. *Blood*, 52(3):499–504, 1978. (Cited on pages 96 and 100.)

[130] M. A. Meyers and K. K. Chawla. *Mechanical Behaviors of Materials.* Prentice Hall, 2 edition, 1999. (Cited on page 38.)

[131] J. P. Mills, L. Qie, M. Dao, C. T. Lim, and S. Suresh. Nonlinear elastic and viscoelastic deformation of the human red blood cell with optical tweezers. *Molecular and Cellular Biomechanics*, 1(3):169–180, 2004. (Cited on pages 68, 105, 106, and 120.)

[132] R. Mittal and G. Iaccarino. Immersed boundary methods. *Annual Review of Fluid Mechanics*, 37:239–261, 2005. (Cited on page 50.)

[133] N. A. Mody and M. R. King. Three-dimensional simulations of a platelet-shaped spheroid near a wall in shear flow. *Physics of Fluids*, 17:113302, 2005. (Cited on page 174.)

[134] N. A. Mody and M. R. King. Platelet adhesive dynamics. Part I: Characterization of platelet hydrodynamic collisions and wall effects. *Biophysical Journal*, 95:2539–2555, 2008. (Cited on pages 119 and 174.)

[135] N. Mohandas and P. G. Gallagher. Red cell membrane: Past, present, and future. *Blood*, 112:3939–3948, 2008. (Cited on page 90.)

[136] F. Momen-Heravi, L. Balaj, S. Alian, A.J. Trachtenberg, F. H. Hochberg, J. Skog, and W. P. Kuo. Impact of biofluid viscosity on size and sedimentation efficiency of the isolated microvesicles. *Frontiers in Physiology*, 3:162, 2012. (Cited on page 59.)

[137] S. Nagrath, L. V. Sequist, S. Maheswaran, D. W. Bell, D. Irimia, L. Ulkus, M. R. Smith, E. L. Kwak, S. Digumarthy, A. Muzikansky, P. Ryan, U. J. Balis, R. G. Tompkins, D. A. Haber, and M. Toner. Isolation of rare circulating tumour cells in cancer patients by microchip technology. *Nature*, 450:1235–1239, 2007. (Cited on pages 153 and 160.)

[138] M. Nakamura, S. Bessho, and S. Wada. Spring network based model of a red blood cell for simulating mesoscopic blood flow. *International Journal for Numerical Methods in Biomedical Engineering*, 29(1):114–128, 2013. (Cited on pages 104 and 110.)

[139] B. Neu and H. J. Meiselman. Depletion-mediated red blood cell aggregation in polymer solutions. *Biophysical Journal*, 83:2482–2490, 2002. (Cited on page 63.)

[140] N.-T. Nguyen, S. A. M. Shaegh, N. Kashaninejad, and D.-T. Phan. Design, fabrication and characterization of drug delivery systems based on lab-on-a-chip technology. *Advanced Drug Delivery Reviews*, 65:1403–1419, 2013. (Cited on page 150.)

[141] S. A. Niederer, E. Kerfoot, A. P. Benson, M. O. Bernabeu, O. Bernus, C. Bradley, E. M. Cherry, R. Clayton, F. H. Fenton, A. Garny, E. Heidenreich, S. Land, M. Maleckar, P. Pathmanathan, G. Plank, J. F. Rodríguez, I. Roy, F. B. Sachse, G. Seemann, O. Skavhaug, and N. P. Smith. Verification of cardiac tissue electrophysiology simulators using an N-version benchmark. *Philosophical Transactions of the Royal Society of London A: Mathematical, Physical and Engineering Sciences*, 369(1954):4331–4351, 2011. (Cited on page 79.)

[142] H. Noguchi and G. Gompper. Dynamics of fluid vesicles in shear flow: Effect of the membrane viscosity and thermal fluctuations. *Physical Review E*, 72(1):011901, 2005. (Cited on page 70.)

[143] National Institute of Biomedical Imaging and Bioengineering, 2017. https://www.nibib.nih.gov/science-education/science-topics/computational-modeling. (Cited on page 1.)

[144] T. Omori, T. Ishikawa, Y. Imai, and T. Yamaguchi. Membrane tension of red blood cells pairwisely interacting in simple shear flow. *Journal of Biomechanics*, 46:548–553, 2013. (Cited on page 63.)

[145] Committee on Frontiers at the Interface of Computing and Biology. *Catalyzing Inquiry at the Interface of Computing and Biology*. National Academies Press, 1st edition, 2005. (Cited on page 194.)

[146] N. Pamme. Continuous flow separations in microfluidic devices. *Lab on a Chip*, 7:1644–1659, 2007. (Cited on page 150.)

[147] W. Pan, B. Caswell, and G. E. Karniadakis. A low-dimensional model for the red blood cell. *Soft Matter*, 6:4366–4376, 2010. (Cited on page 68.)

[148] Y. Park, C. A. Best, K Badizadegan, R. R. Dasari, M. S. Feld, T. Kuriabova, M. L. Henle, A. J. Levine, and G. Popescu. Measurement of red blood cell mechanics during morphological changes. *Proceedings of the National Academy of Sciences: Physics*, 107:6731–6736, 2010. (Cited on pages 72 and 105.)

[149] Y. Park, C. A. Best, T. Kuriabova, M. L. Henle, M. S. Feld, A. J. Levine, and G. Popescu. Measurement of the nonlinear elasticity of red blood cell membranes. *Physical Review E, Statistical, nonlinear, and soft matter physics*, 83(5), 2011. (Cited on page 101.)

[150] P. Pathmanathan and R. A. Gray. Verification of computational models of cardiac electro-physiology. *International Journal for Numerical Methods in Biomedical Engineering*, 30(5):525–544, 2014. (Cited on page 78.)

[151] M. Paulitschke, J. Mikita, D. Lerche, and W. Meier. Elastic properties of passive leukemic white blood cells. *International Journal of Microcirculation, Clinical and Experimental*, 10(1):034011, 1991. (Cited on pages 118 and 119.)

[152] C. S. Peskin. Flow patterns around heart valves: A numerical method. *Journal of Computational Physics*, 10(2):252–271, 1972. (Cited on page 50.)

[153] C. S. Peskin. Numerical analysis of blood flow in the heart. *Journal of Computational Physics*, 25:220–252, 1977. (Cited on page 70.)

[154] D. Pinho, T. Yaginuma, and R. Lima. A microfluidic device for partial cell separation and deformability assessment. *BioChip Journal*, 7(4):367–374, 2013. (Cited on page 117.)

[155] I. V. Pivkin and G. E. Karniadakis. Accurate coarse-grained modeling of red blood cells. *Physical Review Letters*, 101, 2008. (Cited on page 69.)

[156] A. S. Popel and P. C. Johnson. Microcirculation and hemorheology. *Annual Review of Fluid Mechanics*, 37:43–69, 2005. (Cited on page 84.)

[157] C. Pozrikidis. Effect of membrane bending stiffness on the deformation of capsules in simple shear flow. *Journal of Fluid Mechanics*, 440.209–291, 2001. (Cited on page 68.)

[158] C. Pozrikidis. *Computational Hydrodynamics of Capsules and Biological Cells*. Chapman & Hall/CRC Mathematical and Computational Biology. CRC Press, 2010. (Cited on pages 72, 102, 111, 112, and 113.)

[159] I. Proudman and J. R. A. Pearson. Expansions at small Reynolds numbers for the flow past a sphere and a circular cylinder. *Journal of Fluid Mechanics*, 2(3):237–262, 1957. (Cited on page 51.)

[160] M. Puig-de Morales-Marinkovic, K. T. Turner, J. P. Butler, J. J. Fredberg, and S. Suresh. Viscoelasticity of the human red blood cell. *American Journal of Physiology - Cell Physiology*, 19:023301, 2007. (Cited on page 105.)

[161] K. A. Rejniak. Investigating dynamical deformations of tumor cells in circulation: Predictions from a theoretical model. *Frontiers in Oncology*, 2, 2012. (Cited on page 183.)

[162] R. O. Rodrigues, D. Pinho, V. Faustino, and R. Lima. A simple microfluidic device for the deformability assessment of blood cells in a continuous flow. *Biomedical Microdevices*, 17(6), 2015. (Cited on pages 116, 117, and 118.)

[163] P. Saffman and M. Delbruck. Brownian motion in biological membranes. *Proceedings of the National Academy of Sciences*, 72(8):3111, 1975. (Cited on page 103.)

[164] L. Saiz, S. Bandyopadhyay, and M. L. Klein. Towards an understanding of complex biological membranes from atomistic molecular dynamics simulations. *Bioscience Reports*, 22:151–173, 2002. (Cited on page 68.)

[165] Salome. Open-source integration platform for numerical simulation, 2018 (accessed April 23, 2018). http://www.salome-platform.org. (Cited on pages 26 and 141.)

[166] S. M. Santana, H. Liu, N. H. Bander, J. P. Gleghorn, and B. J. Kirby. Immunocapture of prostate cancer cells by use of anti-PSMA antibodies in microdevices. *Biomedical Microdevices*, 14(2):401–407, 2012. (Cited on pages 155, 156, and 163.)

[167] R. G. Sargent. Verification and validation of simulation models. In *Proceedings of the 2011 Winter Simulation Conference*, pages 159–165, 2011. (Cited on pages 77, 80, and 83.)

[168] A. F. Sarioglu, N. Aceto, N. Kojic, M. C. Donaldson, M. Zeinali, B. Hamza, A. Engstrom, H. Zhu, T. K. Sundaresan, D. T. Miyamoto, X. Luo, A. Bardia, B. S. Wittner, S. Ramaswamy, T. Shioda, D. T. Ting, S. L. Stott, R. Kapur, S. Maheswaran, D. A. Haber, and M. Toner. A microfluidic device for label-free, physical capture of circulating tumor cell clusters. *Nature Methods*, 12:685–691, 2015. (Cited on page 153.)

[169] U. D. Schiller. A unified operator splitting approach for multi-scale fluid-particle coupling in the lattice Boltzmann method. *Computer Physics Communications*, 185:2586–2597, 2014. (Cited on page 50.)

[170] S. Schlesinger, R. E. Crosbie, R. E. Gagné, G. S. Innis, C. S. Lalwani, J. Loch, R. J. Sylvester, R. D. Wright, N. Kheir, and D. Bartos. Terminology for model credibility. *Simulation*, 32(3):103–104, 1979. (Cited on page 77.)

[171] T. Shiga, N. Maeda, and K. Kon. Erythrocyte rheology. *Critical Reviews in Oncology, Hematology*, 10(1):9–48, 1990. (Cited on page 84.)

[172] J. Siguenza, S. Mendez, and F. Nicoud. How should the optical tweezers experiment be used to characterize the red blood cell membrane mechanics? *Biomechanics and Modeling in Mechanobiology*, 16(5):1645–1657, 2017. (Cited on pages 76 and 120.)

[173] R. Skalak, A. Tozeren, R. P. Zarda, and S. Chien. Strain energy function of red blood cell membranes. *Biophysical Journal*, 13:245–264, 1973. (Cited on pages 73 and 120.)

[174] M. Slavík, K. Bachratá, H. Bachratý, and K. Kovalčíková. The sensitivity of the statistical characteristics to the selected parameters of the simulation model in the red blood cell flow simulations. In *2017 International Conference on Information and Digital Technologies (IDT)*, pages 344–349, 2017. (Cited on page 123.)

[175] J. P. Smith, T. B. Lannin, Y. A. Syed, S. M. Santana, and B. J. Kirby. Parametric control of collision rates and capture rates in geometrically enhanced differential immunocapture (GEDI) microfluidic devices for rare cell capture. *Biomedical Microdevices*, 16(1):143–151, 2014. (Cited on pages 154, 155, 156, 163, and 164.)

[176] R. Smith. Open dynamics engine. http://www.ode.org, 2017. (Cited on page 136.)

[177] C. Song, P. Wang, and H. A. Makse. A phase diagram for jammed matter. *Nature*, 453:629–632, 2008. (Cited on page 62.)

[178] T. A. Springer. Traffic signals for lymphocyte recirculation and leukocyte emigration: The multistep paradigm. *Cell*, 76(2):301–314, 1994. (Cited on page 178.)

[179] S. L. Stott and et al. Isolation of circulating tumor cells using a microvortex generating herringbone-chip. *Proceedings of the National Academy of Sciences*, 107(43):18392–18397, 2010. (Cited on page 153.)

[180] A. Studer. Modeling red blood cell deformation in a rotary blood pump. Master's thesis, ETH Zurich, 3 2016. ID: 09-923-897. (Cited on page 173.)

[181] D. Suarez. *Change agent*. Dutton, 2017. (Cited on page 192.)

[182] K. Surawathanawises, V. Wiedorna, and X. Cheng. Micropatterned macroporous structures in microfluidic devices for viral separation from whole blood. *Analyst*, 142(12):2220–2228, 2017. (Cited on page 150.)

[183] Y. H. Tang, L. Lu, H. Li, C. Evangelinos, L. Grinberg, V. Sachdeva, and G. E. Karniadakis. OpenRBC: A fast simulator of red blood cells at protein resolution. *Biophysical Journal*, 112:2030–2037, 2017. (Cited on page 76.)

[184] M. E. Taskin, K. H. Fraser, T. Zhang, C. Wu, B. P. Griffith, and Z. J. Wu. Evaluation of Eulerian and Lagrangian models for hemolysis estimation. *American Society for Artificial Internal Organs Journal*, 54(4):363–372, 2012. (Cited on page 169.)

[185] G. K. Thiruvathukal, K. Laufer, and B. Gonzalez. Unit testing considered useful. *Computing in Science and Engineering*, 8(6), 2006. (Cited on page 126.)

[186] G. Tomaiuolo. Biomechanical properties of red blood cells in health and disease towards microfluidics. *Biomicrofluidics*, 8:051501, 2014. (Cited on pages 98, 101, 103, and 237.)

[187] G. Tomaiuolo and S. Guido. Start-up shape dynamics of red blood cells in microcapillary flow. *Microvascular Research*, 82:35–41, 2011. (Cited on page 115.)

[188] R. Tran-Son-Tay, S. P. Sutera, and P. R. Rao. Determination of red blood cell membrane viscosity from rheoscopic observations of tank-treading motion. *Biophysical Journal*, 46(1):65–72, 1984. (Cited on pages 103, 110, 112, and 113.)

[189] K. Tsubota and S. Wada. Elastic force of red blood cell membrane during tank-treading motion: Consideration of the membrane's natural state. *International Journal of Mechanical Sciences*, 52:356–364, 2010. (Cited on pages 70 and 104.)

[190] A. Tsuji and S. Ohnishi. Restriction of the lateral motion of band 3 in the erythrocyte membrane by the cytoskeletal network: Dependence on spectrin association state. *Biochemistry*, 25(20):6133–6139, 1986. (Cited on page 103.)

[191] R. Vernekar, T. Krueger, K. Loutherback, K. Morton, and D. Inglis. Anisotropic permeability in deterministic lateral displacement arrays. *Lab on a Chip*, 17:3318–3330, 2017. (Cited on page 153.)

[192] R. E. Waugh. Surface viscosity measurements from large bilayer vesicle tether formation. II. Experiments. *Biophysical Journal*, 39(1):29–37, 1982. (Cited on page 103.)

[193] R. E. Waugh and E. A. Evans. Thermoelasticity of red blood cell membrane. *Biophysical Journal*, 26:115–132, 1979. (Cited on page 100.)

[194] X. Yang, X. Zhang, Z. Li, and G-W. He. A smoothing technique for discrete delta functions with application to immersed boundary method in moving boundary simulations. *Journal of Computational Physics*, 228(20):7821–7836, 2009. (Cited on page 50.)

[195] T. Ye, N. Phan-Tien, and C. T. Lim. Particle-based simulations of red blood cells - A review. *Journal of Biomechanics*, 49:2255–2266, 2016. (Cited on pages 70 and 71.)

[196] X. Yin and J. Zhang. An improved bounce-back scheme for complex boundary conditions in lattice Boltzmann method. *Journal of Computational Physics*, 231:4295–4303, 2012. (Cited on page 139.)

[197] G. Zavodszky, B. van Rooij, V. Azizi, S. Alowayyed, and A. Hoekstra. Hemocell: A high-performance microscopic cellular library. In *Procedia Computer Science 108C, International Conference on Computational Science, ICCS 2017, 12-14 June 2017, Zurich, Switzerland*, pages 159–165, 2017. (Cited on pages 76 and 130.)

[198] N. F. Zeng and W. D. Ristenpart. Mechanical response of red blood cells entering a constriction. *Biomicrofluidics*, 8(1):ID 064123, 2014. (Cited on page 116.)

[199] Y. Zhai, A. Wang, D. Koh, P. Schneidera, and K. W. Oh. A robust, portable and backflow-free micromixing device based on both capillary- and vacuum-driven flow. *Lab on a Chip*, 18(2):276–284, 2018. (Cited on page 150.)

[200] J. Zhang. Lattice Boltzmann method for microfluidics: Models and applications. *Microfluidics and Nanofluidics*, 10:1–28, 2011. (Cited on page 70.)

Index